nutrition facts

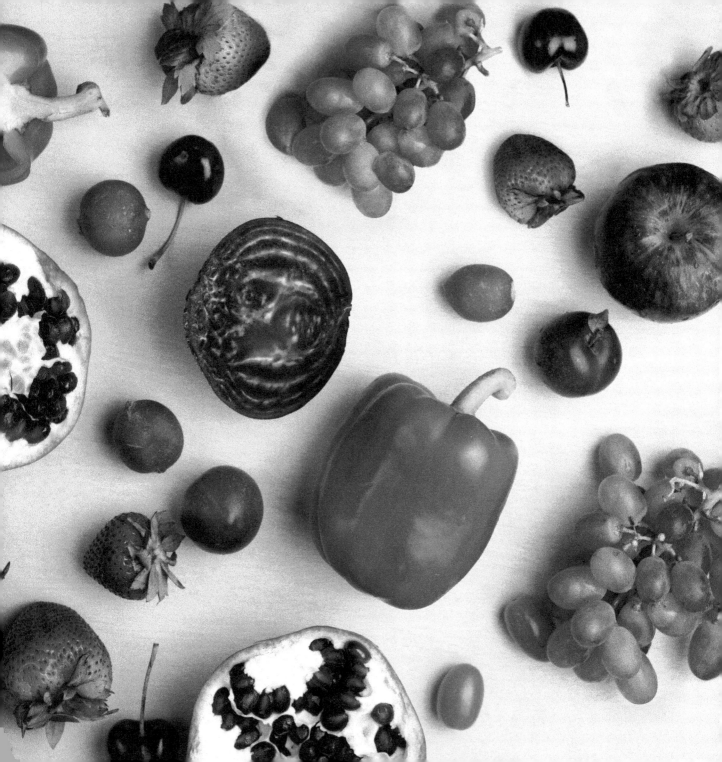

nutrition facts

THE TRUTH ABOUT FOOD

KAREN FRAZIER

ROCKRIDGE
PRESS

Cover photography © Shutterstock/Ana Blazic Pavlovic, Stockfoood/PhotoCuisine/Studio, and Stocksy/Susan Brooks-Dammann; Interior photography © Stocksy/Alita Ong, pages 2, 8, 24, 46, 122, and 162; iStockphoto/Chris Gramly, page 7

ISBN: Print 978-1-62315-611-4
eBook 978-1-62315-616-9

contents

introduction

Hippocrates, the father of medicine, famously said, "Let food be thy medicine, and let medicine be thy food." Even though he lived in the fourth century BCE, Hippocrates was onto something. Since then, physicians, nutritionists, and scientists have offered variations on Hippocrates's statement, the most basic of these being the motto "You are what you eat."

66 In 2010, 12 states had an obesity rate of 30 percent or greater, while an additional 36 states had an obesity rate of 25 percent or higher. 99

While this premise may sound simple, most people may find it complex to apply in real life. Food and drink are a combination of macronutrients—carbohydrates, protein, and fats—that contain a combination of micronutrients such as vitamins and minerals. Humans need these macronutrients and micronutrients to nourish their bodies.

Food is essential to the survival of every species. For humans, though, food provides more than mere sustenance. It has taken on cultural, social, emotional, and even religious significance. Many family and social traditions focus on food and drink. For better or worse, people build a relationship with food, a relationship that often carries a far greater role in one's life than providing simple nutrients to enable survival.

You can't turn on the television and radio or surf the Internet without being inundated with the latest nutritional news. Media outlets breathlessly report which foods might finally allow you to effortlessly lose 20 pounds, prolong your life, protect your heart, or return your youthful glow. The problem is that the results of these studies often seem to contradict one another, and you may be left confused about the best way to optimize your health through food.

Changes in the general state of health for Americans over the past decades are disturbing. Since 1990, obesity in America has grown at an alarming rate. According to the Harvard T. H. Chan School of Public Health, in 1990 nearly every US state had an obesity rate of about 15 percent or

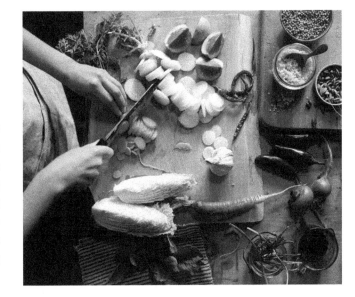

lower. In 2010, 12 states had an obesity rate of 30 percent or greater, while an additional 36 states had an obesity rate of 25 percent or higher. The Centers for Disease Control (CDC) notes that a full one-third of Americans (78.6 million people) are obese. Similar trends are occurring elsewhere throughout the Western world.

Meanwhile, according to the CDC, heart disease and stroke are the first and third top causes of death in the American population, respectively. The National Institute of Allergy and Infectious Diseases at the National Institutes of Health notes in their executive summary that autoimmune diseases are also on the rise in the American public, with autoimmune conditions affecting 5 to 8 percent of the population, or between 14 and 22 million people.

The statistics indicate a population growing sicker with each passing year. What is causing this decline in American health? If you are what you eat, then perhaps the answer lies on the breakfast, lunch, and dinner plates of the American populace.

As Hippocrates suggested so many centuries ago, if you want to begin to heal, then at least part of the cure lies in the foods you eat. This book aims to provide you with the simple, unvarnished truth about nutrition. Using scientific evidence and facts, it will help you begin to understand how different types of micronutrients and macronutrients affect your body, so you can live the healthiest, most vibrant life possible.

> **❝ Let food be thy medicine, and let medicine be thy food. ❞** —HIPPOCRATES

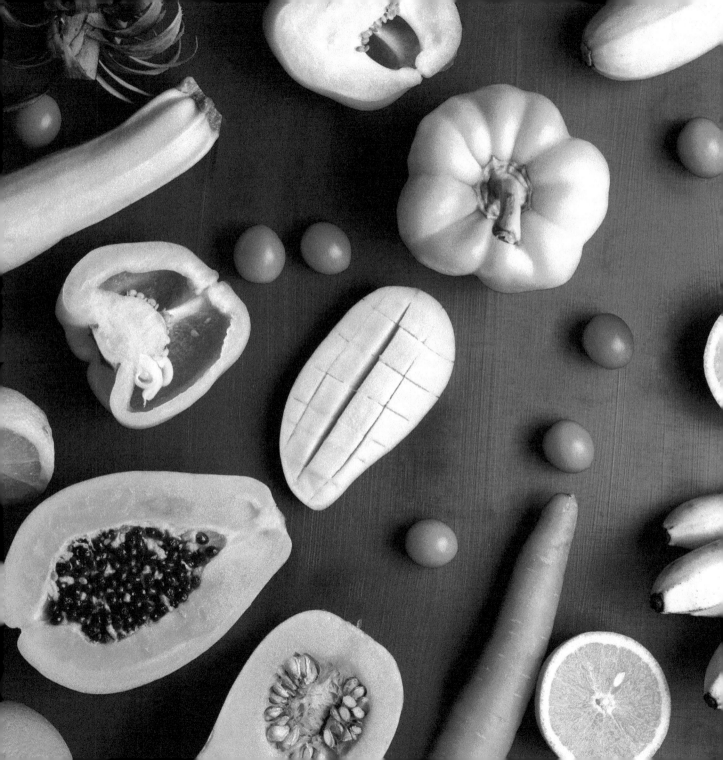

nutrition & health

Just how closely does what you eat correlate to your health? According to the CDC, nutrition and health are intimately connected. Healthful eating can reduce the risk of developing a number of conditions, including osteoporosis, cardiovascular disease, obesity, dental cavities, certain cancers, stroke, and diabetes. Proper nutrition is also essential for the growth and development of children. A multitude of scientific and medical studies continue to demonstrate this close connection between food and health. Clearly, the foods we eat and feed our families play an important role in our health, wellness, and quality of life.

what nutrition is

what nutrition is

Nutrition involves eating healthy, whole foods that meet your body's nutrient needs while supporting good health. Indeed, the World Health Organization defines nutrition as "the intake of food, considered in relation to the body's dietary needs." The study of nutrition examines how food intake affects the body, requiring scientists to look at all aspects of the foods we eat.

Proper nutrition consists of eating the appropriate combination and amounts of whole foods that provide your body with the micronutrients, macronutrients, and phytonutrients it needs to promote good health and protect against disease. These needs may vary from person to person based upon a number of factors such as weight, sex, age, food allergies and sensitivities, activity level, and specific health concerns.

MACRONUTRIENTS

Macronutrients are the components of foods that provide calories (or energy) to the body. There are three main macronutrients:

* Carbohydrates
* Fats
* Proteins

Each of these macronutrients plays an essential role in how the body utilizes and stores energy for basic functions, activities of daily life, and more strenuous activities. See chapter 3 for further information about each of these macronutrients.

MICRONUTRIENTS

Micronutrients are the minute but essential amounts of elements in food that your body needs to sustain function and good health. Vitamins and minerals are examples of micronutrients. While your body needs only small amounts of each vitamin and mineral, overall these micronutrients are vital to every bodily system and process. See chapter 2 for further information about how key vitamins affect different body parts and functions.

PHYTONUTRIENTS

Also called phytochemicals, phytonutrients are found in plant foods. These compounds appear to offer protective benefits against disease in humans. A number of compounds fall into the category of phytonutrients, including flavonoids, phenolic acids, lignans, and stilbenes.

WHOLE FOODS

The most nutritious foods for your body are whole, minimally processed foods. Foods that fall into this category include:

* Fruits and vegetables
* Herbs and spices
* Meat, seafood, fish, and poultry
* Eggs
* Whole, minimally processed grains such as brown rice and buckwheat
* Dairy products
* Nuts, seeds, and legumes

MYTH

If you don't want to get a cold, load up on the vitamin C.

FACT

While evidence shows that vitamin C taken once you have a cold may help to shorten the duration and severity of a cold, taking it as a preventive doesn't work. Vitamin C is still good for you in many other ways, including as an antioxidant, so make sure to make foods rich in vitamin C, such as citrus fruits, a part of your daily diet.

what nutrition isn't

what nutrition isn't

MYTH

You can burn more calories eating certain foods than those foods contain.

FACT

The negative calorie myth is a pervasive one that's been around for years, and it sounds like an easy fix for weight loss. However, if it sounds too good to be true, that's because it is. While it would be great if you could subsist solely on celery or lettuce or grapefruit to lose weight, there is no scientific evidence supporting the idea that some foods have a negative calorie impact. Still, low-calorie fresh fruits and vegetables tend to be high in fiber, so they are a great addition to a healthy diet.

Nutrition isn't eating nutritionally bankrupt foods, and then taking vitamin supplements to get the nutrients your body needs. While vitamins and supplements can provide help during times when your diet isn't optimal, they shouldn't be your go-to method for meeting your body's micronutrient needs.

Unfortunately, busy lives, financial concerns, addictions, and taste preferences can lead one to a diet severely lacking in nutrition, by consuming a diet high in processed foods and fast food, sugar, chemical additives, and empty calories.

PROCESSED FOODS AND FAST FOOD

Processed foods are those that line the middle shelves of the grocery stores. Most frequently, they come in bags, boxes, cans, and packages and have long lists of difficult-to-pronounce ingredients, including additives, preservatives, artificial flavorings and colorings, sugar, high-fructose corn syrup, and chemical thickeners, among others.

Fast food can be healthy if you make the right choices (such as the veggies and fruit at the salad bar), but, in general, fast foods contain high levels of sugar, salt, and processed ingredients.

SUGAR

Sugar comes in many forms, mostly highly refined. Some of the more common forms of sugar include evaporated cane juice, white sugar, brown sugar, high-fructose corn syrup, and corn syrup. According to *Harvard Health*, sugar makes up about 10 percent of the daily caloric intake of most Americans. While it certainly makes food sweeter, sugar may have a number of deleterious effects on human health. A 2014 study published in the journal *JAMA Internal Medicine* showed a correlation between intake of added sugars and risk of all-cause mortality, particularly that from cardiovascular disease.

CHEMICAL ADDITIVES: ARTIFICIAL SWEETENERS, ADDITIVES, PRESERVATIVES, PESTICIDES, AND MORE

While the US Food and Drug Administration (FDA) confers a rating of either "safe" or "generally recognized as safe" on the chemical additives in foods, the truth is that very little is known about the long-term effects of many of these additives. For example, the Harvard T. H. Chan School of Public Health notes that studies into artificial sweeteners show conflicting results—ranging from some benefits, to no effect on health, to deleterious effects.

EMPTY CALORIES

Foods that have "empty calories" are those that give the body energy while meeting few, if any, of the body's micronutrient needs. Sugary drinks like soda are a good example of empty calories, as are refined carbohydrates such as white rice, sugary baked goods, and pasta made from white flour.

MYTH

Omega-6 fatty acids are bad for you, while omega-3 fatty acids are healthy.

FACT

Both omega-6 and omega-3 fatty acids are essential fatty acids, and your body needs an omega-6 to omega-3 ratio of about 1:1 to 2:1. The problem is that the Standard American Diet, which is full of processed foods, is too high in omega-6 fatty acids, creating a ratio of 16:1. This imbalance promotes inflammation. The reason health care providers may recommend supplementing with omega-3 fatty acids is to bring this ratio closer to the optimal one.

historical facts and trivia

historical facts and trivia

* The establishment of the Food and Drug Administration was preceded by that of the Department of Agriculture and the Bureau of Chemistry. Abraham Lincoln created both of these entities in 1862.
* Before 1906, there were no specific laws prohibiting misleading food labels. In 1906, the Pure Food and Drugs Act passed, banning interstate commerce of mislabeled foods and medicines, and providing for inspection of products by the Bureau of Chemistry.
* 1906 was a big year in American food safety. That was the year that Upton Sinclair's book *The Jungle* was published. Although it was a work of fiction, the book exposed the abhorrent practices of the meatpacking industry and led to the 1906 Meat Inspection Act, which reformed the entire industry.
* Ancel Keys, an American physiologist, was the first scientist to formulate the Lipid Hypothesis, which correlated saturated fat and cholesterol intake with heart disease. Keys was also the inventor of the K-ration, which was provided to US military troops.
* Vegetarians and vegans may have difficulty getting enough vitamin B_{12}, because the vitamin is primarily found in animal sources. However, some yeasts, such as nutritional yeast, do contain vitamin B_{12}, making them a good source of this micronutrient for a vegan diet.
* If you enjoy soda and buy the standard 20-ounce bottle, you'll be getting 65 grams of sugar, which amounts to nearly two shot glasses full of sugar.

* According to the US Department of Agriculture (USDA), the American food supply provides about 3,800 calories per day per person, about 800 calories more per day than in the 1950s.
* Dr. Andrew Weil notes that almost 50 percent of Americans get at least a third of their daily calories from junk food.
* According to the Center for Food Safety, about 75 percent of the processed foods in supermarkets contain some genetically modified ingredients. Most of these ingredients are derived from genetically modified corn and soy.
* In 2015, the USDA's Food and Nutrition Service set out new guidelines for healthier school lunches that included more fresh produce, more whole grains, reduced-fat dairy products, and calorie and portion limitations.

MYTH

Eggs are not healthy.

FACT

You can thank a *Time* magazine cover from 1984 featuring two eggs and a slice of bacon making a frown face for the popularization of this myth. While the yolks of eggs do contain cholesterol, the Mayo Clinic notes that the effect of cholesterol from eating a few eggs is negligible. One egg has about 140 mg of cholesterol, mostly in the yolk. Eggs are also high in protein and contain a number of nutrients, including vitamins A, B_6, B_{12}, and D, as well as magnesium and potassium.

how nutrition relates to . . .

how nutrition relates to . . .

MYTH

Spicy foods cause ulcers.

FACT

Spicy foods may aggravate stomach issues such as ulcers or heartburn, but they don't cause ulcers. A large number of ulcers are caused by bacterial infections, and some are caused by lifestyle choices such as smoking, or certain medications. So don't stay away from spicy food because you're afraid of getting an ulcer. However, you may wish to avoid it if you already have one and don't want to aggravate it.

GROWTH

Nutrition for growth and development starts before a baby is even born. What a pregnant mother eats may affect her baby even into his or her adulthood. A 1993 article in the journal *Lancet* explores the link between low birth weight associated with poor fetal nutrition, and the development of adult-onset diabetes and cardiovascular disease later in life. Infants in utero whose mothers are deficient in folic acid are at risk of being born with tube defects, according to the US National Library of Medicine.

The foods that babies, toddlers, and children eat may also affect their growth and development. A 1970 study published in the *New England Journal of Medicine* looked at 19 children hospitalized for undernutrition in their first year. The study showed that these children scored lower in multiple areas of development including height, weight, head circumference, and mental development. Over the past four decades, further studies and reports, including a United Nations Standing Committee on Nutrition report, have borne out those results, consistently showing that children receiving poor nutrition (often due to poverty) don't do as well in school and lag behind in other health markers as well.

REPRODUCTION

Adequate nutrition plays an important role in the reproductive process. Undernourished or anorexic women falling under a certain body weight or body composition may stop ovulating, which in turn affects fertility, according to the journal *Human Reproduction Update*. A 2015 article in *Contemporary OB/GYN* states that ovulation suppression occurs because alterations in body composition due to extreme fat loss hinder gonadotropin secretion, which is what stimulates ovulation. Fat gain results in the return of function to the ovaries.

HEALTH

Your body needs certain amounts of vitamins and minerals for optimal function. To help you meet these nutritional requirements, the USDA has established recommendations for intake of vitamins and minerals, called the Dietary Reference Intake (DRI) or Recommended Dietary Allowance (RDA). Vitamins and minerals support the work that your organs and systems do to maintain health throughout your body. Lack of vitamins and minerals can cause various health conditions, such as scurvy when there is an absence of vitamin C, or rickets when vitamin D is deficient.

METABOLISM

Metabolism refers to how your body uses food intake to meets its energetic needs. The body is very efficient and does everything it can to store energy (as fat) for times of famine. Therefore, when you drastically reduce the amount of food you eat, your body may sense famine and begin to store fat, slowing weight loss or even causing weight gain. In addition, the foods you eat may affect various hormones in your body, which contribute to how well you metabolize and store food.

how nutrition relates to . . . . . .

MYTH

Calories are all that matter for weight loss.

FACT

Calories do matter, but they aren't the only factor in weight loss and gain. Recent research shows that weight loss and gain is far more complex than a simple calories in–calories out formula. Other factors that may play a role include activity levels, hormonal imbalances, and food allergies, among others. While it's important to strive to control portion sizes and not overeat, a balanced diet for a healthy adult is about 2,000 calories per day.

what "healthy" means

what "healthy" means

You may want to be healthy, but what does it mean to be in good health? Is it an absence of illness, or is good health something more?

According to the World Health Organization, "Health is a state of complete physical, mental, and social well-being and not merely the absence of disease or infirmity."

ABSENCE OF DISEASE OR INFIRMITY

Have you ever noticed that two people can be exposed to the same germs, but only one person gets sick? What is the difference between those two people? Often, the reason one person becomes ill while another doesn't has to do with the function of each one's immune system. People with strong immune systems are better able to fight the germs they are exposed to, so that exposure is less likely to lead to illness. People with weaker immune systems may be more prone to developing sickness after exposure to pathogens, because their immune system lacks the ability to kick into gear to fight the bugs.

Other forms of disease, such as heart disease and cancer, are also indicators of poor health. People with chronic illness, such as autoimmune conditions like lupus or lifestyle diseases such as type 2 diabetes, may not be 100 percent healthy, but they can improve their health by controlling symptoms of the disease by adopting lifestyle changes such as better nutrition and exercise.

PHYSICAL WELL-BEING

Physical well-being encompasses a whole host of health markers, including:

* Having the appropriate body composition in terms of height and weight as well as body mass index (BMI)
* Maintaining a healthy diet

- Being able to engage in activities of daily life and recreational activities without pain, discomfort, or undue fatigue
- Having a healthy appearance, including hair, skin, nails, and teeth
- Abstaining from or enjoying only a moderate intake of intoxicants such as alcohol
- Abstaining from illegal and mind-altering drugs
- Seeking appropriate preventive, palliative, and acute care for health issues
- Engaging in adequate physical activity
- Receiving adequate sleep (seven to nine hours per night)
- Managing stress

MENTAL WELL-BEING

Mental and emotional well-being involves engaging in appropriate self-care in order to maintain mental and emotional health. This might include:

- Making time for activities you enjoy
- Being self-aware
- Engaging in stress-releasing activities such as meditation and relaxation
- Expressing yourself emotionally
- Finding ways to engage your mind and intellect in order to keep it flexible and healthy
- Seeking support from friends, family, or professionals during times of mental or emotional stress
- Engaging in hobbies
- Pursuing a satisfying career
- Helping others
- Engaging in spiritual pursuits

MYTH

When you have the option, always choose the low-fat or fat-free versions of foods.

FACT

While lowering fat may be beneficial for saving calories, these foods may be higher in sugar, which comes with its own set of problems. Because fat adds so much flavor to foods, many food manufacturers replace it with sugar when they take out the fat. Sugar increases blood glucose, which causes your body to release insulin. Insulin serves as a fat storage hormone, keeping fat trapped in fat cells and transferring new energy to fat cells for later use.

SOCIAL WELL-BEING

Social well-being occurs when one is able to function comfortably and safely within social groups such as families, groups of friends, work organizations, religious organizations, communities, and society as a whole. Markers of social well-being include:

* Ability to work within a group for mutual common interests or betterment
* Ability to peacefully coexist within a group, family, or society
* Ability to resolve conflicts in a constructive way
* Peaceful and constructive participation in multiple types of social groups, such as friendships, churches, communities, families, and organizations

SAFETY AND SECURITY

Another factor affecting health is your safety and security. If you live in a constant state of insecurity or experience a continued risk to safety, it is difficult to be fully healthy. For example, people who experience food insecurity due to poverty or lack of availability may be less likely to exhibit good health. Living in a constant state of fear or insecurity keeps you in a permanent state of fight-or-flight, which releases stress hormones throughout your body. While these stress hormones are important when you are truly in danger, they quickly dissipate when the danger subsides. However, when you are in a constant state of fear or stress, the hormones remain present, which can cause physical problems.

ACCESS TO SERVICES

Having access to essential services, including healthful foods, reliable shelter, fresh water, and adequate health care, are all critical to good health. Without the ability to access these types of resources regularly, good health can diminish.

food as medicine

Food is very powerful medicine. It affects you on every level, so the quality of the food you consume determines your bodily health. Different foods have varying nutrient profiles, and different nutrients support various bodily organs, systems, and functions. Therefore, the foods you eat can and do affect your health.

ELIMINATING FOODS FOR HEALTH

In some cases, eliminating certain foods can help you find your way to better health. For someone with the autoimmune disorder celiac disease, eating gluten, a protein found in wheat, rye, and barley, causes damage to the small intestines. This damage causes severe pain and blocks the body's ability to absorb nutrients from foods. While there is no cure for celiac disease, eliminating gluten from the diet can control the symptoms, allowing the intestines to heal so they can once again absorb nutrients.

For people with irritable bowel syndrome (IBS), eliminating a group of foods called FODMAPs (see page 185) may help control the symptoms of the disease. Similarly, people with allergies or sensitivities to foods like peanuts or dairy can eliminate these foods from their diets to improve health and decrease bodily inflammation.

EATING FOODS FOR CERTAIN HEALTH CONDITIONS

Some naturopaths and functional medicine specialists recommend certain foods to help various health conditions, but studies remain inconclusive. For example, fermented foods, which are high in enzymes and probiotics, may help people with digestive issues. Someone with anemia may benefit from eating iron-rich and B_{12}-rich foods such as organ meats. A person with a cold may shorten its duration by eating foods rich in vitamin C, such as citrus fruits.

food with medicine

food with medicine

Some foods interact negatively with certain drugs, while other foods may help boost the effectiveness of medication. The FDA notes a number of food-and-drug interactions that may:

* Prevent a medication from working or lessen its effects
* Worsen or improve the medication's side effects
* Interact and cause new side effects

The FDA warns that the medications you take may change the way your body processes and metabolizes the foods you eat.

Some common food-and-medication interactions include the following:

* Taking alcohol with antihistamines and narcotics may increase the effects of sleepiness from these medications. Taking alcohol with narcotics can depress respiration, which can be very dangerous.
* Mixing alcohol with analgesics may cause liver problems.
* Using bronchodilators (asthma medications) with caffeine-containing foods and drinks may increase side effects like rapid heartbeat and heart palpitations.
* Taking ACE inhibitors with high-potassium foods (such as bananas) may cause dangerously high levels of potassium in the body.
* Combining statins with grapefruits or grapefruit juice may cause the level of statins in the body to rise.
* Blood thinners combined with foods that also thin blood, like garlic and ginger, may cause the blood to thin too much.

You can also use foods to enhance wellness when you take certain medications. For example, there is some evidence that niacin can help boost your levels of "good" cholesterol (HDL). Foods high in niacin (vitamin B$_3$) include fish, pork, peanuts, liver, and mushrooms. For people with significant levels of inflammation or autoimmune disease, foods containing omega-3 fatty acids can help reduce inflammation. These foods include fish, flaxseed, chia seeds, and walnuts.

food versus medicine

Eating a healthful diet full of whole foods is essential, but in cases of acute illness, food may be only part of the healing process. When faced with acute illness, some people choose to seek only a nutritional solution while eschewing medicine. This approach is understandable, since food lacks the side effects of medicine. However, in some cases medication is absolutely essential. It is important to work with your primary health care provider to seek a full program for healing. If you do plan to seek a primarily nutritional approach to healing when faced with illness, do so in consultation with a trained professional such as a naturopath.

food versus medicine

MYTH
Alcohol will help you sleep better.

FACT
Alcohol is a central nervous system depressant, so it may help you fall asleep more quickly and sleep pretty deeply for an hour or two, but you won't stay asleep for long. If you do, it won't be a very restful sleep. That's because after the first few hours of boozy sleep, alcohol can induce sleep disturbances that disrupt REM, the most important stage of sleep.

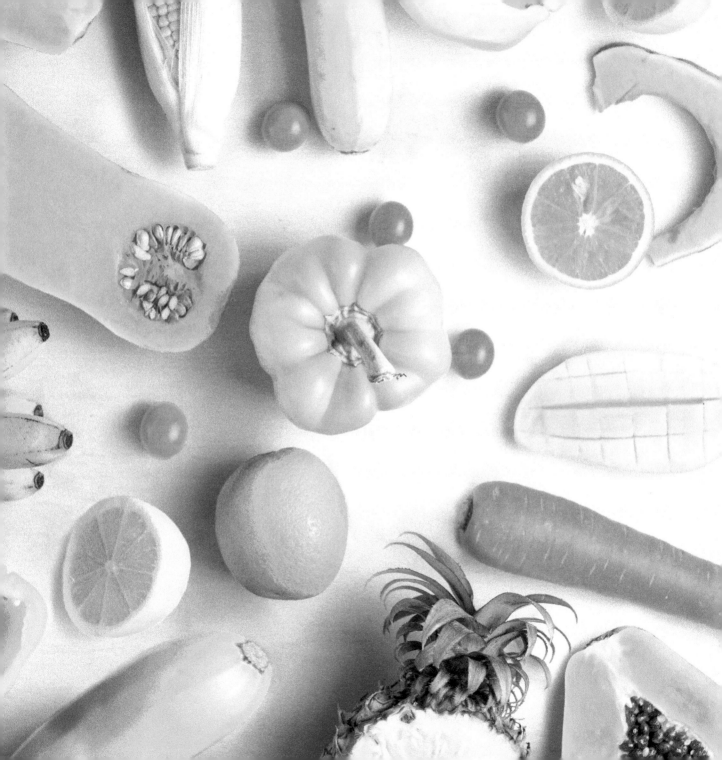

the body

Every organ, system, and body part relies on the fuel you provide it via the foods you eat in order to continue to function properly. While many people tend to think of proper nutrition only in terms of weight loss or weight gain, it is, in fact, crucial to the health of every single cell in your body. This is why it is so important that you forgo foods containing empty calories and instead eat a variety of nutritionally dense foods—those foods that are packed with beneficial elements like vitamins, minerals, phytochemicals, and fiber. Your body relies on these healthful foods to function properly.

THE BODY
digestion

When you take a bite of food or a sip of a beverage, digestion begins as soon as the substance enters your mouth. From there, it takes a long journey through the alimentary canal (digestive tract), making various stops along the way so your body can extract as many nutrients as possible until the unused portions exit through your bowels as waste.

While digestion takes place in the alimentary canal, it is the organs of the digestive system that make it possible. These include the stomach, liver, pancreas, and gallbladder.

When you eat or drink, your body begins to break down the foods and move them through the digestive tract. Digestion begins in the mouth, where chewing and the addition of saliva, which is a digestive juice, break down the starches in the foods you eat. Your teeth also pulverize proteins and fats so they can journey comfortably through the body.

Once you're done chewing, you swallow the food and saliva, and it begins traveling through your esophagus, which uses muscular contractions to move the food through it and into your stomach. In essence, your esophagus merely serves as a passage through which food moves from mouth to stomach.

In the stomach, the food mixes with stomach acid, which breaks down proteins. Next, it moves into your small intestine. There, bile acids from the liver and pancreatic juice from the pancreas mix with the foods to break down fat and further break down starches and proteins. When the breakdown of food is complete in the small intestine, small fingerlike structures on the walls of the intestine called villi absorb the nutrients from the broken-down food and feed them into the bloodstream so they can nourish your body.

Finally, the remainder waste products, now relatively devoid of nutrients, mix with water in the large intestine to form stool. From there, the stool travels into the rectum and exits the body through the anus.

absorption

In order to function properly, your body needs to receive energy (measured as calories) from the foods you eat. It also needs macronutrients like protein and micronutrients like vitamins and minerals for healthy function. If food traveled through your alimentary canal with no absorption, your organs and systems would be unable to operate properly.

The belief many people have that most digestion takes place in the stomach is incorrect. While the stomach supplies acid to break down foods and controls the speed of release of food particles into the small intestine, the only substance the stomach absorbs and feeds into the bloodstream is alcohol. All other nutrient absorption occurs in the small intestines. This takes place after food particles have been broken down into liquid form by mechanical and chemical processes such as chewing and mixing with digestive juices like saliva, stomach acid, pancreatic juice, and bile. Breaking down foods in this manner is very important to the body, because it presents the food particles in such a way that they are now ready to release their nutrients for use in the body.

The small intestine in an adult is about 22 feet long stretched to its full length, but it is so tightly packed together that it fits within your abdominal cavity. The small intestine contains three separate parts: the duodenum, the jejunum, and the ileum. In the duodenum, the broken-down food mixes with bile and pancreatic juices, which contain enzymes to break down food and extract individual nutrients. The jejunum is lined with mucosal folds to increase its surface area in order to optimize absorption. The jejunum also contains small fingerlike projections called villi as well as tightly packed microvilli. These tiny projections absorb the nutrients, passing them through the mucosal folds and into the bloodstream to nourish the body. Finally, the remaining mixture moves into the ileum, where the body reabsorbs the bile acids to be returned to the liver. While most nutrients are absorbed in the jejunum, it is in the ileum where the body absorbs vitamin B_{12} into the bloodstream.

---

absorption

ENERGY

At its most basic level, food serves as a source of energy for your body so it can meet its most basic functions. When you eat food, it can be burned as fuel, converted to glucose and then burned as fuel, or stored in fat cells for later use. If you take in more energy as food than your body needs to function, it will be stored in fat cells for use when it is needed.

THE BODY
metabolism

CALORIES

Many Americans have come to dread the calorie. They really aren't as scary as they seem. Rather, calories are a measure of food energy. Technically a kilocalorie, the definition of a calorie is the amount of energy required to raise the temperature of one gram of water by 1°C. In general, health experts believe that expending more energy than you consume (burning more calories than you eat) results in fat loss, while consuming more than you burn results in fat storage. While this basic tenet provides a rule of thumb for consumption, many other factors figure into weight loss or gain, such as hormones and basal metabolic rate.

You don't eat food just because it tastes good. You also have a biological urge to eat to supply your body with energy. Metabolism is the conversion of food to meet the body's energy needs, and it is a very complex process.

Even if you did nothing all day, your body would require energy to function. Your body uses energy for blood circulation, breathing, body temperature control, digestion and absorption, brain function, and elimination. These are your body's basic functions. The energy it takes for your body to perform these functions is your basal metabolic rate. This is the lowest amount of energy you need to obtain from either food intake or fat stores to survive.

Metabolism of fuel in your body requires chemicals and hormones to convert food or body fat into energy. During the process of digestion, food mixes with digestive juices and is broken down into its energy-containing macronutrients: protein, carbohydrates, and fats. This process releases specific vitamins and minerals for absorption into the body. Macronutrients are further broken down into energy-containing units the body can absorb easily, such as amino acids, glucose (simple sugars), and fatty acids. Once absorbed into the bloodstream, these particles travel to the body's cells, where they are metabolized as energy. If the energy supplied to the body via food (measured as kilocalories, but known simply as "calories") is sufficient to meet the body's energy needs, then all of the food energy is used. If food energy exceeds the body's needs, then the body stores the surplus energy in the fat cells for later use. If food energy isn't sufficient to meet the body's needs, then the body pulls energy from its fat stores.

This is a simplified explanation of metabolism, but the conversion of food to energy can vary significantly from person to person based on a number of factors, including hormonal levels in the body, the age and sex of the person, the amount of lean body mass, and so on.

head

Your head contains a number of important organs and parts, all with their own unique nutritional needs. Of course, the largest and most important organ in the head is the brain, which is covered in more detail on page 41. Along with the brain, your eyes and optic nerves, nose and nasal passages, ears and ear canals, and the mouth, as well as hair growth, all require nourishment.

EYES AND OPTIC NERVES

You've probably heard the old adage that eating carrots improves eyesight, but is it true? Carrots are high in beta-carotene, which converts to vitamin A in the body. According to *Scientific American*, vitamin A allows the eye to convert low light signals, and it helps keep the cornea healthy.

The American Optometric Association also notes that eating a diet high in antioxidants can help with visual health by reducing the risk of eye diseases. These vitamins and antioxidants may include the following:

LUTEIN AND ZEAXANTHIN

These two nutrients are carotenoids, which are pigments found in vegetables. They are present in dark, leafy greens such as kale, chard, and spinach, as well as in eggs and other foods. Various studies, such as one published in the April 2004 *Journal of the American Optometric Association*, show that adequate consumption of these nutrients can help reduce the risk of developing age-related macular degeneration.

VITAMIN C AND VITAMIN E

The American Optometric Association notes that a body of research shows that consumption of vitamins C and E, which are antioxidants, can help reduce the risk of developing cataracts. Vitamin C is present in a number of plant foods, such as citrus fruits and strawberries.

ESSENTIAL FATTY ACIDS

The eyes need essential fatty acids for eye health, particularly the omega-3 fatty acids DHA and EPA. The American Optometric Association states that these two forms of omega-3 fatty acids are essential for proper retinal function and visual development. You can find omega-3 fatty acids in fatty fish such as salmon and mackerel, as well as in walnuts and seeds such as chia and flax.

ZINC

The eye contains a high concentration of zinc, which assists the liver in providing vitamin A to the retina. Studies also show a correlation between zinc deficiency and visual impairments such as cataracts and night blindness. Zinc is a mineral present in dairy products, eggs, beef, pork, and seafood.

EARS

A study in the 2013 *International Journal of Audiology* showed that a strong relationship exists between adequate nutrition and better hearing (lack of hearing loss). According to the Life Extension Foundation, certain nutrients may help prevent hearing loss or improve tinnitus (ringing in the ears), including:

* Antioxidants, found in an array of fruits and vegetables
* Carnitine, an amino acid found in animal proteins
* Lipoic acid, an antioxidant found in red meat, cruciferous vegetables, and organ meats
* Folate, a B-complex vitamin found in legumes and dark leafy greens
* Vitamin B_{12}, found in animal proteins and nutritional yeast
* Magnesium, a mineral found in dark leafy greens, fish, nuts and seeds, and bananas
* Melatonin, a hormone found naturally in foods such as bananas, avocados, milk, and oatmeal
* Coenzyme Q_{10}, a vitamin-like substance found in broccoli, nuts, and seafood

- Omega-3 fatty acids, an essential fatty acid found in seafood, nuts, and seeds
- Taurine, an amino acid found in animal protein and nutritional yeast

NOSE

Your nose and sinuses are often the first place allergies, sensitivities, or intolerances to foods show up. These and other chronic and acute illnesses can lead to sinus inflammation, which results in an excess of mucus, sinus pain and pressure, and/or blocked sinuses.

Discovering the source of any sensitivities and eliminating them, as well as eating an anti-inflammatory diet high in nutrients like omega-3 fatty acids and antioxidants, can help keep sinuses clear and free of pressure.

MOUTH

The American Dental Association recommends a nutrient-dense diet containing a balance of vitamins and minerals for optimal mouth health. Some nutrients especially essential for healthy teeth and gums include:

- Calcium
- Magnesium
- Vitamin D
- Protein
- Phosphorus
- Vitamin C
- Vitamin A

HAIR

Healthy hair requires a number of vitamins and minerals, including iron, B-complex vitamins, zinc, and vitamin D.

AGING

Have you ever wondered why, as people grow older, their bodies and appearance change so significantly? As you age, your cells reproduce at a slower rate, which accounts for many of the signs of aging, such as slower healing and loss of cognition. Your skin loses collagen, which in turn causes a loss of elasticity. The body produces less melanin, so hair loses pigment and turns gray. Another source of aging is oxidative stress. Eating foods that contain antioxidants can help slow or reduce oxidative stress.

chest, stomach & back

chest, stomach & back

Your thoracic (chest) and abdominal cavities contain the majority of your body's organs, including your heart and lungs. Maintaining healthy breasts and back is also essential for good health.

HEART

Scientific studies have shown a very strong correlation between diet and heart health. The American Heart Association recommends a calorie-moderated heart-healthy diet emphasizing nutrient-dense foods such as fruits and vegetables, whole grains, low-fat dairy products, poultry, fish, and nuts. The organization also recommends minimizing sugar, sodium, red meat, and other foods high in saturated fats. The AHA recommends limiting fats to about five percent of daily calories and limiting the cholesterol in foods you eat.

Along with heart-healthy food recommendations, another important consideration in nourishing your heart is electrolytes. These minerals, which include sodium, potassium, calcium, magnesium, and bicarbonate, control the heart's electrical impulses. They are required in proper balance to maintain healthy heart function.

A 1:1 to 2:1 balance of omega-6 to omega-3 fatty acids is also necessary (see page 186). The American Heart Association recommends eating fish and seafood several times per week in order to reduce inflammation, which studies have shown to correlate to heart disease, and improve the ratio of omega-3 to omega-6 fatty acids into a more beneficial range.

LUNGS

Your lungs drive your body's respiratory system, providing oxygen for the blood to carry to your cells. The American Lung Association's recommendations for a lung-healthy diet are similar to those of the AHA for a healthy heart.

An article in the April 2004 *Journal of Tuberculosis and Lung Disease* examined the effect of nutrition on lung disease and noted that anti-oxidants such as vitamins C, E, and A, carotenoids, and minerals like magnesium, zinc, manganese, and selenium can help fight oxidative stress that leads to lung disease and have proven beneficial for maintenance of lung health.

BREASTS

In the United States, breast cancer is the most common type of cancer in women. The CDC notes that in 2011 more than 220,000 women and 2,000 men received a breast cancer diagnosis, while nearly 41,000 women and 500 men died of the disease. It is possible to use a healthy diet to maintain breast health, in an effort to prevent the development of breast cancer.

Recommendations for nutrition to minimize the risk of developing breast cancer include the following:

* Eat a diet that contains between 10 and 20 percent of your calories from fat.
* Minimize consumption of animal proteins. Instead, focus on getting your protein from plant sources such as soy, or by combining plant foods to make a complete protein.
* On a daily basis, eat six servings of healthy whole grains, three to five servings of vegetables, two to four servings of fruit, one to two servings of legumes, and one to two servings of soy.
* Stay hydrated.
* Limit or eliminate caffeine, alcohol, nitrates, and food additives.

BACK

If you've ever suffered back pain, then you know how debilitating it can be. While many solutions for a healthy back involve exercise, stretching, and posture, nutrition can also affect your back.

Electrolytes are essential in controlling muscle contraction and relaxation. An electrolyte imbalance can cause muscular spasm, which can lead to back pain.

The Cleveland Clinic notes that a number of foods can cause or aggravate inflammation, which can lead to back pain. Other foods may help minimize the risk of back pain, including those that keep bones healthy and strong and allow you to remain hydrated. To that end, the clinic recommends a diet for back pain that includes the following:

* Minimizing red meats and saturated fats
* Minimizing processed foods and simple carbohydrates such as sugar and white rice
* Consuming a moderate amount of red wine (about 4 ounces three or four times per week)
* Eating fish at least three times per week
* Eating plenty of fresh fruits and vegetables
* Eating foods high in calcium, such as low-fat dairy products and dark leafy greens
* Drinking eight 8-ounce glasses of water daily

arms & legs

Your legs carry you everywhere, while your arms help you carry out important tasks. You may not typically think in terms of nutrition for your arms and legs, but when you consider how necessary they are to daily activity, it's easy to see why nourishing them is important. Arms and legs consist of muscles, bones, fat, nerves, and skin.

BONES

Your bones do much more than just provide musculoskeletal support. They also produce red blood cells, which grow within the marrow of your bones for about seven days before they are released into your bloodstream. There they make up approximately 45 percent of blood volume and serve to circulate oxygen and nutrients throughout the body, in addition to carrying carbon dioxide back to the lungs for reoxygenation.

With such important functions, maintaining bone health is vitally important. As the American Academy of Osteopathic Surgeons explains, the nutrients calcium and vitamin D are essential for building and maintaining healthy bones. When there isn't enough calcium in the diet, the body removes what it needs from the bones. Chronic calcium deficiency can lead to weakening of the bones, which can result in the bones becoming fragile, a condition known as osteoporosis. This fragility may cause fractures in the arms, legs, or anywhere else in the body where the bones have been weakened.

When children don't have sufficient vitamin D in their diets, they develop a condition called rickets, which is a softening and weakening of the bones in the legs. In adults, vitamin D deficiency can result in osteomalacia, a softening of the bones that can cause deformities in the long bones of the arms and legs.

arms & legs

ENDURANCE

Endurance is different from strength, but it is equally important. Endurance refers to how well you can sustain an activity over time. Building endurance involves engaging in progressively longer sessions of activity. This allows your muscles, connective tissue, heart, and lungs to let you go a little further and a little longer each day.

The body's primary source for vitamin D is sunlight, which it absorbs into the skin and converts to vitamin D. People in northern or cloudy climates, or those who spend most of their time indoors, may be at risk of vitamin D deficiency. To counteract this, you can drink milk fortified with vitamin D, which works synergistically with vitamin C to strengthen the bones.

In order to facilitate red blood cell production in the bone marrow, you need to consume adequate amounts of iron, vitamin B_{12}, and vitamin B_6. If you are deficient in iron or red blood cells, you are at risk of developing anemia, a condition that leads to weakness, fatigue, paleness, and sometimes heart palpitations. Eating iron- and vitamin B–rich foods such as red meat can help you build healthy red blood cells.

NERVES

Nerves run throughout your body, ultimately connecting to your spinal cord, which sits protected inside your spinal column. The spinal cord carries signals back and forth between the nerves and the brain. Nerve impulses from the brain arriving via the spinal cord allow you to move your arms, legs, hands, and feet. They also alert your brain when you experience a pain-causing injury.

Many nutrients affect your nerves. Consuming adequate amounts of vitamins B_1, B_6, and B_9, found in animal proteins and dairy products, can protect you from developing nerve illnesses that affect the hands, arms, and legs, including beriberi and peripheral neuropathy. Vitamin E, found in almonds, wheat germ, and milk, helps the nerves carry signals to your limbs and extremities.

MUSCLES

Your skeletal muscles contract and relax, allowing movement in your arms and legs. Muscle strength and endurance are essential for these functions, because they allow you to perform heavy duties over extended periods.

Protein is found in each of your body's cells, but it is especially important in building muscle. Your body synthesizes dietary protein into muscle tissue. You can find protein in animal foods as well as plant sources such as soy.

Another important nutrient for muscle function is electrolytes (see page 111). Maintaining a proper balance of electrolytes will keep your arm and leg muscles contracting and relaxing as needed, and will help you avoid uncomfortable cramping. Anyone who has ever had a painful nighttime calf cramp understands what an electrolyte imbalance can cause. These cramps are typically caused by low levels of the electrolyte mineral potassium, found in bananas and potatoes.

arms & legs

WORKOUTS

Not surprisingly, exercising requires more energy than not exercising. Therefore, regular workouts are a great way to increase your body's energy (caloric) requirements. Workouts can help in two ways. First, a workout will burn extra energy. Second, as you increase muscle mass via your workouts, your body experiences a very slight boost in basal metabolic rate. Working out regularly can improve your quality of life, providing you with strength, endurance, and flexibility, as well as increased energy.

organs & muscles

organs & muscles

CELL REPRODUCTION

Your body is continuously making new cells. Cell reproduction occurs when a cell splits in two or more pieces, making exact copies of itself. Cell reproduction is responsible for creating healthy new tissue, as in wound healing. Proper nutrition is essential for cell reproduction. Providing your body with adequate nutrition gives the cells what they need to divide and reproduce.

Your organs are the engines of your body. It is within your organs that your body's most vital functions are carried out, from neural function in your brain to digestion in your stomach, hormonal production in your thyroid and pancreas, and circulation and respiration in your heart and lungs, to name a few.

SKIN

The skin is the body's largest organ. It is one of the first places to show the effects of poor nutrition, which can manifest as acne, inflammation, rashes, hives, and other issues. According to the Linus Pauling Institute at Oregon State University, the nutrients most essential for healthy skin are vitamins A, C, D, and E, flavonoids, and essential fatty acids.

GLANDS AND ORGANS OF THE ENDOCRINE SYSTEM

The endocrine system produces and regulates hormones throughout the body. Hormones play key roles in a wide array of bodily functions, such as reproduction, sleep, hunger and satiation, libido, aging, metabolism, and many others. Organs and glands of the endocrine system include the thyroid, pancreas, parathyroid, adrenal glands, hypothalamus, pineal gland, ovaries, testes, and thymus.

Vitamin D, synthesized from sunlight and found in fortified dairy products, is an essential hormonal regulator within the endocrine system, so consuming adequate levels is necessary for endocrine health.

Cholesterol is an essential component in hormone creation throughout the body. Consuming moderate amounts of dietary cholesterol, found in animal proteins, can also help with hormone balancing and creation. Antioxidants such as vitamins C, E, and A can help keep hormones balanced by preventing or reversing oxidative stress.

Certain foods contain goitrogens, which make thyroid hormone production more difficult, so people with hypothyroid issues should consume them only in moderation. Goitrogenic foods include cruciferous vegetables, soy, mustard greens, pears, sweet potatoes, and horseradish, among others.

URINARY SYSTEM ORGANS

The organs of your urinary system consist of your kidneys and bladder. Your kidneys filter waste from the blood and then turn it into urine. The bladder collects the urine and stores it until you excrete it. Both the kidneys and bladder can become infected if bacteria enter the urinary tract through the urethra and travel through the ureters. Sometimes dietary issues, such as a very high-protein diet or a diet high in purines, can cause painful kidney stones.

The National Kidney Foundation recommends the DASH diet (see page 159) for overall kidney health and for reducing the risk of developing kidney stones.

DIGESTIVE SYSTEM ORGANS

The digestive system is made up of several organs: the liver, stomach, gallbladder, pancreas, liver, small intestine, and large intestine. Proper nutrition can help minimize the symptoms of digestive diseases:

* People with celiac disease, an autoimmune disorder affecting the small intestine, can minimize symptoms by completely eliminating gluten from the diet.
* People with irritable bowel syndrome (IBS) may experience symptom relief by following a diet that eliminates certain types of carbohydrates called FODMAPs (see page 185). Monash University created the low-FODMAP diet, and you can find information about FODMAPs on their website.
* People experiencing acid reflux (heartburn) or gastroesophageal reflux disease may be able to eliminate symptoms by removing acidic foods—those with a pH of 5 or less—from their diet, lowering fat intake, eating smaller meals, and eliminating spicy foods.

STRENGTH

How strong you are is determined by how much of a load you can push, pull, lift, or lower. You build strength through a combination of progressive resistance, such as weight lifting, and a healthy diet that contains plenty of protein to build muscle. When you lift, lower, push, and pull heavy loads, your muscles sustain small tears. Resting for 48 hours or longer allows the proteins you eat to heal those muscles, making them slightly larger and slightly stronger than they were before. If you continue to increase the volume of the object you push, pull, lift, or lower, allowing adequate time for healing in between, over time you will gain strength.

MUSCLES

Your body has three types of muscles: skeletal, cardiac, and smooth (organ). Skeletal muscles are voluntary—you control their movement. Cardiac and smooth muscles are involuntary. Because electrolytes are so important in all muscle contraction and relaxation, your body has multiple mechanisms in place to keep electrolytes in balance. Hormones control how the body stores and concentrates electrolytes to keep them within the necessary range. If you consume too much salt, your body retains water in order to keep the sodium diluted to maintain proper concentration. It's also the reason that eating salty foods makes you thirsty—so you'll drink fluid to counter the sodium concentration.

To help maintain electrolyte balance, it is recommended that you drink about 64 ounces of water daily and eat foods that contain potassium, magnesium, calcium, and sodium. If you sweat excessively during a workout session or high heat, your body will lose electrolytes in your sweat. Replenish them through a healthy diet or by consuming a sugar-free electrolyte sports drink such as coconut water.

brain

The brain is your body's central processing unit, controlling all bodily functions, both voluntary and involuntary. It is constantly at work, sending signals throughout the body via the spinal cord and nerves.

Because this organ is so essential for so many processes in the body, it requires a great deal of your energy intake and stores, in spite of occupying only 2 percent of your body mass. According to *Scientific American*, the brain accounts for about 20 percent of the body's total energy usage on a daily basis. A majority of this energy usage goes to the firing of neurons to send signals throughout the body. This makes the brain the body's biggest user of energy. Because of this, the brain has a number of nutritional needs.

GLUCOSE

Your brain and nervous system need glucose for fuel. Neurons are the cells of the brain and nervous system that carry signals and messages back and forth between the body and the brain. Because neurons can't store glucose on their own, they must get them from supplies of glucose in the bloodstream. Glucose, or blood sugar, comes from consumption of simple and complex carbohydrates, as well as from the synthesis of proteins.

Complex carbohydrates are the most consistent and efficient form of glucose to fuel your brain. Because they contain complex sugars and often fiber, the body absorbs them more slowly into the bloodstream, which ensures steady delivery of glucose to the brain. Simple carbohydrates raise blood sugar rapidly, causing the pancreas to release insulin quickly into the bloodstream. Insulin is a hormone that reduces blood sugar levels by moving the fuel that the blood glucose provides into storage. It also controls the release of stored fuel from the fat cells into the bloodstream for immediate use. When the body releases a large amount of insulin, it stores the fuel instead of putting it to immediate use. When this happens, there is less fuel available for the brain to do its work.

brain

BRAINPOWER

The foods you eat can boost your brainpower! Eating a diet low in sugar and high in nutrient-dense foods can help you stay alert, keep your neurotransmitters balanced, and even ward off cognitive diseases such as Alzheimer's and dementia. Boost your brainpower by eating a nutrient-dense, varied diet low in sugars and processed foods and high in healthy plant foods and fish. Make sure you get plenty of omega-3 fatty acids as well, to balance your fatty acid profiles.

MEMORY

You are who you are because of your memories. You are the sum total of all experiences you've had. Memory is important, not just because it defines you as a human being, but also because it allows you to build on things you have learned in the past so you can continue to grow and change. Protect your memory by eating foods high in omega-3 fatty acids, such as fish and walnuts. Avoid sugar and minimize alcohol to keep your memory humming along as you age.

PROTEIN

The body uses amino acids from the protein you eat to make neurotransmitters, or other brain chemicals that enhance or inhibit brain function. Different amino acids have differing effects on the brain. For example, tryptophan has a light sedating effect on the brain, while tyrosine stimulates it.

Because of the brain's use of amino acids, you need to have protein in your diet. Good sources of protein include meat and poultry, dairy products, soy, and plant combinations that together make a complete protein, such as rice and beans.

FAT

About two-thirds of your brain volume consists of fat. Brain neurons have layers of fatty acid molecules in their cell membranes, which come from the fat in your diet. Neurons are also protected in a myelin sheath, which is mostly made up of fatty acids. Along with providing protection for neurons, your brain also requires fatty acids, particularly omega-3 and omega-6 fatty acids, to make long-chain fatty acids used in cell membranes. Fatty acids also assist in the release of neurotransmitters, as well as in cognitive function.

Omega-3 and omega-6 fatty acids are often called essential fatty acids (EFAs) because, while your body needs them, it does not produce them on its own. Instead, you need to get these EFAs from dietary sources such as plant and animal foods. EFAs are so important to the brain that some medical studies link low EFA levels to diseases such as depression, Alzheimer's, and Parkinson's.

CHOLESTEROL

Because cholesterol is closely correlated with heart disease, many people believe that foods containing cholesterol should be completely avoided. In fact, your body needs cholesterol, which is naturally produced in the liver.

Cholesterol is essential for brain function. Approximately 25 percent of the body's cholesterol is used to help build membranes in the brain and assist in the synthesis of important substances like vitamin D, cortisol, and sex hormones. A 2008 study published in the *American Journal of Geriatric Psychiatry* showed that elderly individuals with the highest levels of cholesterol also had the highest levels of cognitive function. A 2013 study conducted at the University of California at Davis demonstrated that high levels of HDL ("good" cholesterol) and low levels of LDL ("bad" cholesterol) appeared to provide a protective benefit against the development of Alzheimer's.

While consuming excessive quantities of dietary cholesterol is certainly not recommended for heart health, there are dietary approaches to improving HDL while decreasing LDL:

* Choose foods high in soluble fiber, such as oatmeal, bran, and vegetables.
* Eat plenty of fish, seafood, and other foods high in omega-3 fatty acids.
* Enjoy extra-virgin olive oil in moderation.
* Cut back on saturated fats and eliminate trans fats.
* Include plenty of fresh fruits, vegetables, and whole grains in your diet.

FLAVONOIDS

Flavonoids have been shown to improve blood flow to the brain, which can help provide fuel and improve cognitive function.

Flavonoids are polyphenol phytonutrients. They have antioxidant properties, and also help fight inflammation. You can find them in red wine, chocolate, apples, tomatoes, bananas, blueberries, cherries, raspberries, and many other plant foods.

VITAMINS

According to an article in the *Natural Review of Neuroscience,* the brain needs an array of vitamins for proper functioning. Rather than popping a pill, the best source of vitamins is a natural one: the foods you eat. Obtaining vitamins mostly from supplements doesn't nourish your body in the same way and, in some cases, may even be toxic.

VITAMIN E

Research at Oregon State University in 2015 showed that low levels of vitamin E increased the risk of developing Alzheimer's disease. You can get more vitamin E in your diet by eating avocados, almonds, and sunflower seeds.

B-COMPLEX VITAMINS

Your brain needs B-complex vitamins for good health. According to an article in the December 2010 issue of the journal *Nutrition Review*, deficiencies in folate and vitamins B_6 and B_{12} correlated with reduced cognitive function. All types of animal proteins are excellent sources of B-complex vitamins.

VITAMIN D

According to the Vitamin D Council, low blood levels of vitamin D correlate with a higher risk of developing cognitive impairment. Vitamin D has protective benefits for the brain, including reducing the risk of developing brain diseases, regulating immunities, and decreasing toxins in the body. Fatty fish and cod liver oil are the best food sources of this vitamin.

If you live in a low-sun climate or don't spend much time in the sun, then supplementation may be a good choice for you. Before relying on vitamin D supplements, discuss your vitamin D status with your primary health care provider to avoid potential toxicity.

VITAMIN C

Vitamin C works in the brain in an antioxidant capacity. It also assists in a number of brain functions such as collagen production. Studies show it provides a protective benefit against stroke and Alzheimer's disease. Good dietary sources of vitamin C include cantaloupe, citrus fruits, and kiwis.

CHOLINE

Choline plays an essential role in normal brain function. While it can be made in the liver, you can also get it from dietary sources, such as quinoa, soy, and cruciferous vegetables.

Choline is particularly important in the developing brain, so pregnant women should consume a diet rich in this nutrient. According to a 2004 study in the *Journal of the American College of Nutrition*, adequate choline during pregnancy can improve lifelong memory for the fetus.

BETA-CAROTENE

Beta-carotene, an antioxidant that converts to vitamin A, may boost long-term cognitive development, according to the Physicians' Health Study II. The study followed men over the short term and long term and discovered that those with long-term beta-carotene supplementation scored much better on cognition than their counterparts, who received a placebo.

brain

MINERALS

A number of minerals may also provide protective benefits in the brain. The best way to make sure you get enough of these trace elements is to eat a variety of foods rather than relying on supplementation.

SELENIUM

Selenium deficiency can suppress or alter hormone production. Foods high in selenium include Brazil nuts, brown rice, chia seeds, and shiitake mushrooms.

CALCIUM

Eating a diet with adequate calcium may provide protection against development of Alzheimer's disease. Calcium deficiency has been linked with some forms of mental illness.

ZINC

Zinc is essential for brain development and neurotransmission. Low consumption of zinc during pregnancy correlates with nervous system abnormalities in the fetus, according to an article in the journal *Biological Psychiatry*. Foods high in zinc include shellfish, red meat, and legumes.

IRON

Iron serves as a cofactor in neurotransmitter synthesis. It also plays a key role in transporting oxygen to the brain. Foods high in iron include organ meats, shellfish, red meat, and dark leafy greens.

COPPER

Copper plays a key role in a number of brain functions. Copper also protects against Alzheimer's disease, Parkinson's disease, and other illnesses. Foods high in copper include dark leafy greens, summer squash, and asparagus.

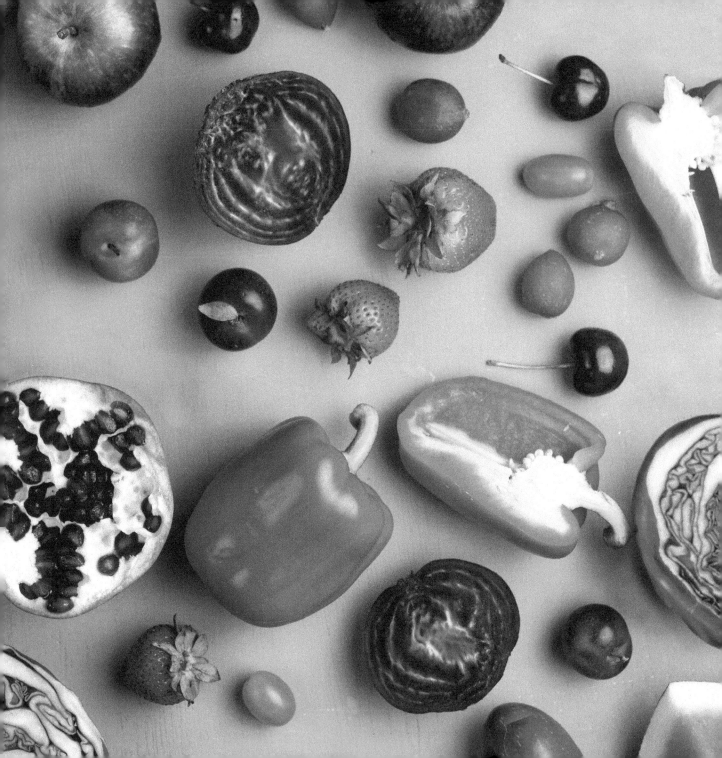

nutrients

The nutritional needs for a healthy diet can vary by age and for women who are pregnant or lactating. Daily nutrient amounts can be considered as a percentage of daily total energy intake (calories) or as specific quantities, and can differ somewhat among the various recommending agencies and organizations. Many of the recommended amounts offered in this section come from the National Institutes of Health, an agency of the US Department of Health and Human Services; the USDA; or the Institute of Medicine (IOM), an independent nonprofit organization that is part of the US National Academies. The IOM provides guidelines for a Recommended Dietary Allowance (RDA) or, where not enough evidence is available, an Adequate Intake (AI).

carbohydrates

Carbohydrates are the main source of fuel for the body. With approximately 4 calories of energy per gram, carbohydrates come in two forms: simple and complex.

Simple carbohydrates are either monosaccharides (consisting of one sugar molecule) or disaccharides (two sugar molecules). Glucose is the most plentiful monosaccharide, while sucrose and lactose are the most common disaccharides.

Complex carbohydrates contain multiple sugar molecules. They include oligosaccharides (three to ten sugar molecules linked into chains) and polysaccharides (chains of up to thousands of sugar molecules). Oligosaccharides are mostly indigestible by humans, acting as a prebiotic, meaning that they feed the "good" bacteria in the gut. Polysaccharides are classified as either starch (digestible) or fiber (indigestible) and are highly beneficial to the body.

THE ROLE OF CARBOHYDRATES

The primary role of carbohydrates is to provide the body with energy. The digestive system breaks down carbohydrates, converting them to glucose. The cells in the body then burn the glucose to produce a molecule called adenosine triphosphate (ATP), which regulates the storage and release of energy from cells.

Insulin, which is secreted in the pancreas, acts as an energy storage hormone. Insulin prompts the use of glucose to meet the body's energy needs or to be stored in the form of body fat. So, if more carbohydrates are consumed than are needed, the resulting glucose will be stored as fat.

Simple carbohydrates can be absorbed so quickly that insulin cannot be released efficiently enough to return blood glucose levels to a desirable level, creating spikes in blood sugar levels. Complex carbohydrates take longer to digest than simple carbohydrates, making them less likely to cause dramatic spikes in blood sugar.

Any excess glucose is converted to glucagon. The body stores about 400 g (1,800 calories) of glucagon in the liver and muscles for later use, in case glucose levels drop too low. The stored energy is then released into the blood to balance blood sugar levels.

DEFICIENCY

When your body is deficient in carbohydrates, it will turn to fats and even proteins for energy. Burning fat without glucose results in a condition known as ketosis, in which ketones are released into the blood. A small amount of ketone in the blood is normal and may even be beneficial. However, in people with type 1 diabetes, a high level of ketones in the blood may lead to ketoacidosis, a life-threatening condition in which the pH of the blood becomes overly acidic. The body will resort to burning muscle tissue (protein) for fuel only in the absence of adequate energy from other sources.

EXCESS

Eating too many simple carbohydrates increases the risk of obesity and type 2 diabetes, and contributes to many other health concerns. While consuming complex carbohydrates tends to be beneficial, some people may have issues of carbohydrate intolerance. People who are sensitive to gluten or who lack enzymes such as lactase, which breaks the bond of the milk sugar lactose, can suffer from an immune response that damages the lining of the small intestine, produces unpleasant symptoms, and causes malabsorption of nutrients.

RECOMMENDED AMOUNTS AND FOOD SOURCES

In addition to energy, carbohydrates also supply the body with a variety of vitamins, minerals, phytonutrients, and antioxidants. The carbohydrates in your diet should mostly be complex carbohydrates, which are found in high-fiber foods such as fruits, vegetables, beans, legumes, and grains. You can also have a serving or two of simple carbohydrates from whole, natural, unprocessed foods such as fruit or dairy products. Try to limit your intake of simple carbohydrates from products that contain sugar.

The USDA recommends that carbohydrates make up 45 to 65 percent of the daily calories for older children and adults, which is about 130 g in a 2000-calorie daily diet.

---

carbohydrates

RDA: CARBOHYDRATES

The RDA varies for each age group:

0 to 6 months	60 g (AI)
7 to 12 months	95 g (AI)
1 year and older	130 g
Pregnant females	175 g
Lactating females	210 g

SUPERFOOD: QUINOA

Like kale, this nutty grain is everywhere right now, earning props from nutritionists. In fact, quinoa is pretty nutritious. For a grain, it contains a lot of protein. It's also very high in fiber, and contains potassium, calcium, iron, vitamin B_6, and magnesium. It also contains a moderate amount of fat. Quinoa comes in many varieties, and it's a great whole-grain substitute for empty carbs like white rice or potatoes.

fats

Fats (lipids) contain mixtures of fatty acids crucial for a healthy body. Fatty acids can be saturated or unsaturated. All fats are composed of chains of carbon atoms with attached hydrogen atoms. The carbon atoms of a saturated fat are attached with a single bond, whereas an unsaturated fat has carbon atoms attached with double bonds. Within unsaturated fats, there are two categories: a monounsaturated fatty acid has only one double bond, while a polyunsaturated fatty acid has more than one.

OMEGA-6 AND OMEGA-3

Two essential fatty acids are linoleic acid (omega-6 fatty acid) and alpha linoleic acid (omega-3 fatty acid). These essential fatty acids must come from food because the body cannot make them. Omega-6 fatty acids are important for cell growth, brain development, and nerve message transmission. Omega-3 fatty acids, including ALA, EPA, and DHA, are crucial for maintaining a healthy heart, ameliorating inflammatory diseases, reducing bad cholesterol, and promoting brain development.

THE ROLE OF FAT

Fat is not absorbed easily in the stomach, thereby making you feel full longer. When the fat reaches the intestine, the gallbladder releases bile, an emulsifier that allows fat to mix with water and enzymes to break it down into fatty acids and glycerol. The fatty acids are either used to make the lipoproteins that carry fats throughout the body, or are stored in fat cells to use as energy.

Fats have many functions in the body:

* Help regulate blood sugar
* Transport hormones and fat-soluble vitamins, such as vitamins A, D, E, and K, throughout the body
* Produce hormones, such as testosterone and estrogen

FAT CONTENT IN OILS

Pure oils all contain about the same amount of fat. However, what varies is the content in saturated, unsaturated, trans, and polyunsaturated fats. Oils high in saturated fat include butter, lard, coconut oil, and palm oil. Oils high in trans fats include margarine and shortening. Oils high in polyunsaturated fats include soybean oil, corn oil, and sunflower oil. Oils highest in monounsaturated fats include olive oil, canola oil, peanut oil, safflower oil, and sesame oil.

* Insulate the body
* Promote a healthy brain, which is 60 percent fat
* Provide a source of immediate and stored energy
* Supply essential nutrients for cell function and repair

DEFICIENCY

Your body needs dietary fat for a number of important functions, including utilization of fat-soluble vitamins. Unfortunately, since the 1960s, dietary guidelines have recommended reducing fat in the diet significantly. However, recent research shows that dietary fat is not necessarily the health threat that was once believed—and may even be beneficial. Because of this, the proposed 2015 Dietary Guidelines for Americans removes restrictions on dietary fat and saturated fat intake. Diets very low in fat tend to be higher in sugar and carbohydrates, which may pose other health threats as well. Likewise, when you remove fat from the diet or severely restrict it, you are more likely to be hungrier or experience cravings because fat is so satiating. Therefore, fat is an essential component of your diet. Choose healthy, natural fats such as those found in animal proteins, butter, extra-virgin olive oil, and coconut oil, among others. Avoid trans fats, which have been linked to heart disease and other health issues.

In addition, while the Western diet tends to be high in fat, it is deficient in omega-3 fatty acids. Omega-3s are found in foods such as fatty fish, Brussels sprouts, kale, salad greens, and some vegetable oils, such as soybean and canola oil. Deficiency in this fatty acid can lead to insulin resistance, metabolic abnormalities, and fatty liver disease.

EXCESS

Too much dietary fat may represent a health danger. Trans fats (partially hydrogenated fats found mostly in processed foods) are strongly linked to heart disease. Fat is calorically dense (9 calories per gram), and consuming too much may cause weight gain. Eating fat itself, however, doesn't necessarily make you fat unless you consume more food energy than your body requires on a regular basis. The type of fat you eat is also important. Recent research suggests that natural saturated fats, found in meat, eggs, and coconuts, are not the devil that medical science once believed.

fats

RDA: FATS

There is no RDA for fat intake, but the Centers for Disease Control and the IOM offer the following guidelines, broken down by age:

1 to 3 years	30 to 40% of total calories
4 to 18 years	25 to 35% of total calories
19 years and older	20 to 35% of total calories

SUPERFOOD: SALMON

Salmon is delicious, and it's really good for you. The pink flesh is relatively high in fat (for a fish), but it's also high in healthy omega-3 fatty acids. Wild-caught salmon is also relatively free of toxins, and it isn't at risk of high mercury concentration. Salmon is also high in vitamin D and serves as an excellent source of protein, so it's the perfect fish for your recommended two to three weekly servings of seafood.

CHOLESTEROL

Recent research has shown that what doctors once thought affected serum blood cholesterol may not be quite right. People with heart disease and high cholesterol were instructed to reduce saturated fat in the diet to help control cholesterol levels. However, recent research suggests that saturated fat doesn't have the effect on blood cholesterol it was once thought to have. Niacin may help control high cholesterol levels, as can eating plant-based foods and getting plenty of exercise.

The proposed 2015 Dietary Guidelines for Americans acknowledges that consuming saturated fats appears to have little correlation in the development of heart disease or cholesterol levels in the blood. Therefore, the guidelines no longer recommend severe limits on dietary intake of saturated fats, except in relation to overall caloric intake and weight gain.

RECOMMENDED AMOUNTS AND FOOD SOURCES

Consuming the recommended amounts of fat can have numerous health benefits:

* Decrease your risk of heart disease and type 2 diabetes
* Help prevent belly fat
* Protect against irregular heartbeat
* Improve good cholesterol levels and blood pressure
* Help prevent plaque buildup in the arteries
* Strengthen the immune system
* Promote healthy skin
* Improve satiation and keep you from getting hungry

Many foods contain fats, such as meats, fatty fish, avocados, olives, nuts, seeds, dairy products, whole grains, oils, and even fruits and vegetables.

proteins

Proteins are composed of long chains of amino acids and are present in every cell in the body. Cells in the digestive tract, however, cannot absorb anything bigger than one or two connected amino acids, called peptides. Digestive enzymes are required to break up the long chains into individual amino acids. Once the peptides are absorbed, enzymes in the cells use the amino acids to build new proteins. This process, called protein synthesis, releases other elements used by the body. The leftover carbon, oxygen, and hydrogen from this process are converted to glucose and used for energy. The nitrogen residue (ammonia) is transported to the liver and converted to urea, which makes urine.

The body uses protein quickly, requiring a consistent supply from food sources. Your body needs 22 different amino acids to create all the proteins it needs, 10 of which must come from food sources. These 10 are called essential amino acids. Your body makes the remaining 12 amino acids.

THE ROLE OF PROTEIN

The proteins in the body have unique tasks:

* Proteins such as keratin and collagen give strength and structure to hair, nails, skin, bones, and teeth.
* Enzymes are made using about half of your dietary protein. Enzymes are the catalysts for the complex reactions in the body.
* Antibodies are blood proteins in the immune system that neutralize and attack invaders in the body such as bacteria and viruses.
* The outer and inner membranes of all cells contain protein that helps move nutrients and waste to and from every part of the body.
* Hormones are chemicals that carry messages around the body. Insulin and glucagon are well-known protein hormones that regulate blood sugar.

RDA: PROTEINS

The RDA varies by age group:

0 to 6 months	9.1 g (AI)
7 to 12 months	11 g
1 to 3 years	13 g
4 to 8 years	19 g
9 to 13 years	34 g
Males 14 to 18 years	52 g
Males 19 years and older	56 g
Females 14 years and older	46 g
Pregnant and lactating females	71 g

* Minerals and proteins keep the body fluid level in balance. Proteins attract water and are too big to pass through membranes, so they maintain the correct amount of fluid in the blood.
* The brain needs a constant supply of glucose to function, so when no energy is available from carbohydrates and fat, the body takes protein from the muscles and other tissues.
* Protein is negatively charged, allowing it to pick up hydrogen atoms (positive charge) when the blood is too acidic, or release them if the blood is too alkaline. This allows the body to maintain a very precise pH.
* Ferritin is a protein that is the main storage form of iron in the body, holding 4500 iron molecules per protein molecule.

DEFICIENCY

Protein deficiency from poor-quality protein or limited intake can cause water retention, impaired immunity, hair loss, muscle wasting, anemia, and liver damage. Protein deficiency is rare in the United States, but pregnant or lactating women, vegetarians, endurance athletes, and people recovering from an injury or surgery could be at risk.

EXCESS

Dangerous levels of protein in the body occur when protein intake is greater than 35 percent of daily calories consumed. Excessive protein can increase the risk of osteoporosis, cancer, weight gain, elevated blood sugar, kidney stones, and gout.

RECOMMENDED AMOUNTS AND FOOD SOURCES

Animal-based proteins, such as meat, poultry, fish, seafood, dairy products, and eggs, provide all 10 essential amino acids. With the exception of soy and quinoa, plant-based proteins are incomplete; no one protein source contains all 10 essential amino acids. Plant foods, then, must be combined to create a complete protein. The current USDA recommendations suggest that for older children and adults, between 10 and 35 percent of their daily calories come from protein. With 1 gram of protein providing 4 calories, that means that adult females require about 46 grams, while adult males require 56 grams.

vitamins

VITAMIN A

Vitamin A is a group of fat-soluble compounds crucial for many functions in the body. The majority of the vitamin A in the body is stored in the liver as retinyl esters. There are two types of chemicals in this group.

PREFORMED VITAMIN A

Retinoids are fat-soluble compounds (retinol, retinoic acid, and others) that are found in animal sources. The body can use these preformed types of vitamin A right away.

PROVITAMIN A

Provitamins are substances that the body converts into vitamins. Carotenoids are a source of provitamin A. Of the more than 500 different carotenoids, about 10 percent are considered to be vitamin A sources, the most important of which is beta-carotene.

Vitamin A is often associated with healthy vision, because the vitamin is a component of a protein in the eye that allows people to see in the dark or in low light. Vitamin A can also slow the development of age-related macular degeneration. Vitamin A also provides these important functions:

* Boosts immune function
* Keeps the skin soft and elastic
* Moistens mucous membranes
* Supports the growth of bones and teeth
* Promotes cell growth
* Maintains the heart, kidneys, and lungs

DEFICIENCY

Vitamin A deficiency is relatively rare in the United States, but in other parts of the world this deficiency is one of the main causes of preventable blindness in children. One of the first symptoms of a vitamin A deficiency is night blindness (xerophthalmia), impaired vision in low light or darkness. Other symptoms of vitamin A deficiency are:

Vitamins are organic compounds necessary for growth and development in the human body. They are required in the human diet in small quantities, because the body cannot make them on its own.

RDA: VITAMIN A

Most adults should get between 50 and 60 percent of the daily RDA for vitamin A from five servings of fruits and vegetables. The estimated average requirements of vitamin A suggested by the IOM varies for each age group:

0 to 6 months	400 mcg
7 to 12 months	500 mcg
1 to 3 years	300 mcg
4 to 8 years	400 mcg
9 to 13 years	600 mcg
Males 14 years and older	900 mcg
Females 14 years and older	700 mcg
Pregnant females up to 18 years	750 mcg
Pregnant females 19 years and older	770 mcg
Lactating females up to 18 years	1,200 mcg
Lactating females 19 years and older	1,300 mcg

* Dry, rough skin
* Slow wound healing
* Reduced capability to sweat
* Impaired sense of smell and taste
* Nerve damage
* Dry mucous membranes
* Impaired reproductive function
* Reduced resistance to respiratory illness

Groups that are at a higher risk of developing a vitamin A deficiency include premature infants, people with cystic fibrosis, vegans, and people with certain gastrointestinal diseases, as well as children, infants, and pregnant and lactating women in developing countries.

EXCESS

Too much vitamin A can cause serious issues because it is fat soluble, which means the excess is stored in the liver and may eventually cause liver damage. Usually, hypervitaminosis (excess vitamin A) is caused by large quantities of vitamin A supplements, not the vitamin A found in one's diet. Long-term excess through chronic use can result in bone pain, fatigue, hair loss, decreased appetite, dry skin, irritability, diarrhea, and reduced growth in children, as well as an increased risk of osteoporosis and bone fractures. Acute excess can lead to increased intracranial pressure, nausea, headaches, blurred vision, skin irritation, vomiting, dizziness, pain in the joints, coma, and even death. Excess preformed vitamin A can cause congenital birth defects such as cleft lip, so pregnant women should consult their doctor before using supplements.

RECOMMENDED AMOUNTS AND FOOD SOURCES

Vitamin A is found in many foods. Preformed vitamin A comes only from animal sources, whereas provitamin A sources include both animal and plant foods. Vitamin A sources include beef liver, fish oils, milk, yogurt, cheese, salmon, eggs, leafy green vegetables, fortified cereals, sweet potato, carrots, broccoli, cantaloupe, pumpkin, bell peppers, mangos, black-eyed peas, and squash.

VITAMIN B

Vitamin B comprises a group of water-soluble vitamins that are essential for converting carbohydrates into usable energy and metabolizing fats and proteins. There are eight B vitamins, each of which plays a unique role in healthy body function.

VITAMIN B$_1$ (THIAMINE)

Vitamin B$_1$ is also known as thiamine or thiamin. It is essential for the formation of adenosine triphosphate (ATP), which the cells use for energy. It also helps strengthen the immune system.

DEFICIENCY
Deficiencies in thiamine may lead to a number of conditions, including dementia, Wernicke-Korsakoff syndrome, beriberi, and cataracts. Thiamine supplementation may also be indicated in patients with heart failure.

RECOMMENDED AMOUNTS AND FOOD SOURCES
Thiamine is found in a number of food sources, including pork, legumes, organ meats, and whole grains.

VITAMIN B$_2$ (RIBOFLAVIN)

Riboflavin is an antioxidant vitamin that helps counteract the effects of the free radicals that form as a result of oxidative stress in the body. It also works synergistically with other B vitamins including folate and vitamin B$_6$, converting them to usable forms. Along with vitamins B$_{12}$ and B$_5$, riboflavin helps the body produce red blood cells.

DEFICIENCY
Deficiencies in vitamin B$_2$ may cause a host of symptoms, such as eye problems and light sensitivity, sores in the corners of the mouth, and a swollen tongue. Supplementation may help with conditions such as cataracts and migraine headaches.

vitamins

RDA: VITAMIN B$_1$

The IOM recommends the following amounts of thiamine:

0 to 6 months	0.2 mg (AI)
7 to 12 months	0.3 mg (AI)
1 to 3 years	0.5 mg
4 to 8 years	0.6 mg
9 to 13 years	0.9 mg
Males 14 years and older	1.2 mg
Females 14 to 18 years	1.0 mg
Females 19 years and older	1.1 mg
Pregnant and lactating females	1.4 mg

RDA: VITAMIN B$_2$

The IOM recommends the following amounts of riboflavin:

0 to 6 months	0.3 mg (AI)
7 to 12 months	0.4 mg (AI)
1 to 3 years	0.5 mg
4 to 8 years	0.6 mg
9 to 13 years	0.9 mg
Males 14 years and older	1.3 mg
Females 14 to 18 years	1.0 mg
Females 19 years and older	1.1 mg
Pregnant females	1.4 mg
Lactating females	1.6 mg

RDA: VITAMIN B$_3$

The IOM recommends the following amounts of niacin:

0 to 6 months	2 mg (AI)
7 to 12 months	4 mg (AI)
1 to 3 years	6 mg
4 to 8 years	8 mg
9 to 13 years	12 mg
Males 14 years and older	16 mg
Females 14 years and older	14 mg
Pregnant females	18 mg
Lactating females	17 mg

Riboflavin comes from a number of food sources, including whole grains, wheat germ, almonds, organ meats, spinach, mushrooms, broccoli, and wild rice.

VITAMIN B$_3$ (NIACIN)

Vitamin B$_3$ has several different names, including nicotinic acid and niacin. It also comes in multiple forms, including niacinamide, nicotinamide, and inositol hexanicotinate. Vitamin B$_3$ has multiple functions in the body, including hormone production and aiding circulation.

DEFICIENCY

Deficiencies in vitamin B$_3$ may cause symptoms such as heartburn, canker sores, and fatigue, as well as a condition called pellagra. Symptoms of pellagra include dementia, diarrhea, and dry, cracked skin.

Vitamin B$_3$ supplementation may be used in treating a number of symptoms. One of its most well-known uses is in improving blood lipid profiles. Some studies have shown that vitamin B$_3$ in the form of niacin can lower unhealthy cholesterol levels. Niacin has also been shown to slow the progression of atherosclerosis, preventing fatty deposits from building up on artery walls.

RECOMMENDED AMOUNTS AND FOOD SOURCES

Niacin is available from a number of food sources, including salmon, beef liver, peanuts, tuna, and sunflower seeds. Likewise, the body can convert the amino acid tryptophan into niacin, so eating meat, poultry, eggs, and dairy can also boost niacin levels.

VITAMIN B$_5$ (PANTOTHENIC ACID)

Vitamin B$_5$ plays several roles in the body, working synergistically with other B vitamins. For example, it works with vitamin B$_2$ and vitamin B$_{12}$ in red blood cell formation, and it helps the body use the other B vitamins.

Deficiencies of this vitamin may lead to symptoms such as insomnia, fatigue, and upper respiratory infections.

RECOMMENDED AMOUNTS AND FOOD SOURCES

Vitamin B_5 supplementation may help improve blood lipid profiles, lowering LDL ("bad") cholesterol and triglycerides while raising HDL ("good") cholesterol. It may also help control symptoms of rheumatoid arthritis and aid in wound healing. Foods high in B_5 include avocados, brewer's yeast, corn, cauliflower, kale, organ meats, sweet potatoes, mushrooms, tomatoes, and oily fish such as trout, salmon, and tuna. Adults need between 1.3 and 1.6 mg of vitamin B_5 daily.

VITAMIN B_6 (PYRIDOXINE)

Pyridoxine is essential for the production of neurotransmitters, which are necessary for normal nerve function. It also plays an important role in brain function, helping produce hormones such as serotonin, melatonin, and norepinephrine.

DEFICIENCY

Deficiencies may cause symptoms such as depression, difficulty concentrating, memory loss, and nervousness.

Supplementing vitamin B_6 may help lower blood homocysteine levels. High homocysteine levels seem to play a role in the development of heart disease. Supplementing B_6 may also help calm morning sickness, prevent depression and PMS, and lower the risk of developing macular degeneration.

RECOMMENDED AMOUNTS AND FOOD SOURCES

For most people, a well-rounded diet should provide a sufficient amount of vitamin B_6. Good dietary sources of pyridoxine include chicken, turkey, oily fish, shrimp, cheese, lentils, spinach, carrots, sunflower seeds, and whole-grain flour.

vitamins

RDA: VITAMIN B_5

The University of Maryland Medical Center recommends the following amounts of pantothenic acid:

0 to 6 months	1.7 mg (AI)
7 to 12 months	1.8 mg (AI)
1 to 3 years	2 mg
4 to 8 years	3 mg
9 to 13 years	4 mg
14 years and older	5 mg
Pregnant females	6 mg
Lactating females	7 mg

RDA: VITAMIN B_6

The University of Maryland Medical Center recommends the following amounts of pyridoxine:

0 to 6 months	0.1 mg (AI)
7 to 12 months	0.3 mg (AI)
1 to 3 years	0.5 mg
4 to 8 years	0.6 mg
9 to 13 years	1.0 mg
Males 14 to 50 years	1.3 mg
Males 51 years and older	1.7 mg
Females 14 to 18 years	1.2 mg
Females 19 to 50 years	1.3 mg
Females 51 years and older	1.5 mg
Pregnant females	1.9 mg
Lactating females	2.0 mg

RDA: VITAMIN B₇

There isn't enough scientific evidence for an RDA of biotin. Instead, the IOM established the adequate intake guidelines as follows:

0 to 6 months	5 mcg
7 to 12 months	6 mcg
1 to 3 years	8 mcg
4 to 8 years	12 mcg
9 to 13 years	20 mcg
14 to 18 years	25 mcg
19 years and older	30 mcg
Pregnant females	30 mcg
Lactating females	35 mcg

RDA: VITAMIN B₉

There isn't enough scientific evidence for an RDA of folic acid. Instead, the IOM established the adequate intake guidelines as follows:

0 to 6 months	65 mcg
7 to 12 months	80 mcg
1 to 3 years	150 mcg
4 to 8 years	200 mcg
9 to 13 years	300 mcg
14 years and older	400 mcg
Pregnant females	600 mcg
Lactating females	500 mcg

VITAMIN B₇ (BIOTIN)

Vitamin B₇ is also known as biotin or vitamin H. This vitamin is especially essential during pregnancy because it supports growth of the embryo.

DEFICIENCY

Deficiency may cause loss of appetite and poor fetal growth. There aren't many studies on biotin, but there is some evidence that supplementation may support healthy growth of hair and nails, reduce the incidence of cradle cap, and improve peripheral neuropathy symptoms.

RECOMMENDED AMOUNTS AND FOOD SOURCES

You can find biotin in tree nuts, whole grains, mushrooms, and bananas.

VITAMIN B₉ (FOLIC ACID)

Also known as folate, folic acid plays important roles in the body, including healthy brain function, fetal development, and mental health. It is also essential for the development of RNA and DNA, as well as red blood cells and tissue growth.

DEFICIENCY

Folic acid is especially important during pregnancy, because folic acid deficiencies can cause neural tube abnormalities and other birth defects. Deficiencies can also cause gum inflammation, brain fog, and poor growth. Likewise, supplementing may provide protective benefits for the heart, prevent age-related deficiencies such as hearing loss and macular degeneration, and may prevent depression.

RECOMMENDED AMOUNTS AND FOOD SOURCES

Folic acid comes from a number of dietary sources including legumes, whole grains, avocados, and salmon.

VITAMIN B$_{12}$ (COBALAMIN)

This is one of the most important B vitamins. It plays a key role in DNA and RNA development, helps form healthy blood cells, provides energy, and controls homocysteine levels in the blood.

DEFICIENCY

Vitamin B$_{12}$ deficiencies may cause a number of symptoms and conditions including anemia, nerve damage, and shortness of breath.

Along with treating pernicious anemia, vitamin B$_{12}$ supplements may be used to reduce homocysteine levels in the blood, to treat fatigue, and to prevent macular degeneration.

RECOMMENDED AMOUNTS AND FOOD SOURCES

Vitamin B$_{12}$ is available primarily in animal-based food sources, particularly meat, poultry, fish, organ meats, and dairy products. Vegetarians, as well as the 10 to 30 percent of adults over 50 who may have difficulty absorbing the vitamin through food, may need to supplement their vitamin B$_{12}$ intake. Children need between 0.9 mcg and 1.8 mcg, and adults need between 2.4 and 2.8 mcg of vitamin B$_{12}$ daily.

RDA: VITAMIN B$_{12}$

The IOM recommends the following amounts of cobalamin:

0 to 6 months	0.4 mcg (AI)
7 to 12 months	0.5 mcg (AI)
1 to 3 years	0.9 mcg
4 to 8 years	1.2 mcg
9 to 13 years	1.8 mcg
14 years and older	2.4 mcg
Pregnant females	2.6 mcg
Lactating females	2.8 mcg

PREGNANCY

Pregnant women have different nutritional needs. Because of the importance of folic acid in fetal development, pregnant women need to eat foods rich in this nutrient, such as spinach, asparagus, oranges, and legumes. Pregnant women need 600 mcg of folic acid daily. Likewise, it is important to eat foods high in calcium, vitamin D, lean protein, and iron. Many obstetricians recommend taking a prenatal multivitamin, which can help improve nutritional status and provide appropriate nutrition for your developing baby.

SMOKING

Smoking may have an effect on the foods you eat. First, smoking dulls the taste buds, so food may taste different, which can affect how much you eat. It also affects your sense of smell, which may influence your enjoyment of food. Smoking has appetite-dampening effects as well. This may lead to malnourishment. It also affects your body's ability to absorb essential nutrients, which may affect your nutritional status as well as your energy levels.

VITAMIN C (ASCORBIC ACID)

Vitamin C is an essential water-soluble vitamin. It is an antioxidant that fights free radicals, and the body uses it for a number of important functions.

ANTIOXIDANT

Vitamin C is a powerful antioxidant that fights the effects of oxidative stress in the body. It helps repair or prevent damage from free radicals, which can cause aging and tissue degeneration in addition to playing a role in a number of conditions, including cancer and heart disease, among others.

CANCER

According to the National Institutes of Health's National Cancer Institute, some studies show that high-dose supplementation of vitamin C may slow reproduction of cancerous cells for certain types of cancer, including prostate, pancreatic, colon, and liver cancers. Other animal studies have shown that the vitamin may block tumor growth in different types of cancers such as sarcoma, mesothelioma, and liver, prostate, and ovarian cancers. However, caution with such therapies is advised, because the FDA does not approve high-dose IV administration of vitamin C for treatment of cancer, and there is some evidence that high doses of vitamin C may block the effectiveness of chemotherapy.

COMMON COLD

For years, common wisdom has suggested that vitamin C supplementation can help prevent the common cold. Unfortunately, no scientific evidence exists to support this adage. However, some studies have shown that vitamin C supplementation may reduce the duration of a cold by about one day.

HEART DISEASE

Studies on how vitamin C affects heart disease have produced mixed results. While vitamin C doesn't appear to have any effect on altering blood lipid profiles, it nonetheless seems to minimize the buildup of plaques that block artery walls and potentially cause heart attacks. It may do this via its antioxidant properties.

SCURVY

Long-term vitamin C deficiency can manifest in a disease called scurvy. Weakness, weight loss, and lethargy, as well as swollen gums, loose teeth, poor wound healing, spontaneous bleeding, and other symptoms characterize scurvy. Eating foods that contain adequate amounts of vitamin C will prevent the disease.

TISSUE GROWTH AND REPAIR

The body uses vitamin C for tissue growth and repair. It is essential in the formation of collagen, a protein the body uses to make healthy tendons, ligaments, blood vessels, and skin. Likewise, vitamin C plays an essential role in wound healing and scar tissue formation, as well as the maintenance and repair of bones, teeth, and cartilage.

DEFICIENCY AND TOXICITY

Studies currently show no correlation between vitamin C supplementation and lowered risk of heart attack or stroke. However, people with low levels of vitamin C are at higher risk of heart attack, stroke, and peripheral artery disease. While it appears that supplementation won't reverse these processes, eating adequate levels of foods containing vitamin C throughout your life may prevent these issues from occurring in the first place.

Because vitamin C is a water-soluble vitamin, there is little chance of developing toxicity. Instead, any excess is excreted in the urine. Most studies indicate that even high doses of vitamin C are safe. When taking high doses of vitamin C orally, though, you may experience diarrhea if you increase your dosage too quickly. Taken over time, your bowel tolerance to the supplement will improve.

RECOMMENDED AMOUNTS AND FOOD SOURCES

If you eat a healthy diet full of foods containing vitamin C, then supplementation is unnecessary. You can find vitamin C in brightly colored fruits and vegetables. Foods that are particularly high in vitamin C include red bell peppers, oranges, grapefruit, kiwis, broccoli, strawberries, and Brussels sprouts.

It is recommended that smokers get an extra 35 mg of vitamin C daily.

vitamins

RDA: VITAMIN C

Dietary reference intakes for vitamin C are as follows:

0 to 6 months	40 mg
7 to 12 months	50 mg
1 to 3 years	15 mg
4 to 8 years	25 mg
9 to 13 years	45 mg
Males 14 to 18 years	75 mg
Males 19 years and older	90 mg
Females 14 to 18 years	65 mg
Females 19 years and older	75 mg
Pregnant females up to 18 years	80 mg
Pregnant females 19 years and older	85 mg
Lactating females up to 18 years	115 mg
Lactating females 19 years and older	120 mg

FAT-SOLUBLE VITAMIN SUPPLEMENTATION

Fat-soluble vitamins (vitamins A, D, E, and K) are stored in the body, and it is possible that they can build up to toxic levels. It's best to try to get your fat-soluble vitamins from eating healthy foods. If you do choose to supplement any of the fat-soluble vitamins, work closely with your health care practitioner.

VITAMIN D

Vitamin D is a fat-soluble vitamin. While it is present in a few foods, most of the vitamin D the body receives is synthesized from the sun.

BONES

Vitamin D works with calcium to promote absorption of this important mineral. Because it enables calcium absorption, vitamin D is essential for bone health. Without it, bone mineralization does not occur, which can lead to a weakening of bones and teeth commonly referred to as rickets in children or osteomalacia in adults. Vitamin D is also important in the prevention of osteoporosis, a weakening of the bones that may occur in older adults.

CANCER

According to the National Institutes of Health's National Cancer Institute, there is evidence showing that individuals living in lower latitudes that enjoy greater sun exposure have a lower incidence of death from certain types of cancer. More research is needed to determine whether this is the result of increased vitamin D synthesis or some other factor. Some studies have shown that maintaining adequate levels of vitamin D may have a protective effect against pancreatic, prostate, colorectal, and breast cancers, but more research is required.

HEART DISEASE

Studies are ongoing into the correlation between vitamin D deficiency and heart disease. However, many studies do show that a deficiency in vitamin D may increase the risk of heart attack, stroke, congestive heart failure, and peripheral artery disease.

IMMUNE SYSTEM

Vitamin D deficiency also appears to play a role in the development of autoimmune diseases in which the body attacks its own tissue. Likewise, deficiency correlates to an increased susceptibility to developing illnesses and diseases.

NERVOUS SYSTEM

Vitamin D plays key roles in your brain and nervous system, helping to maintain normal function and prevent diseases such as amyotrophic lateral sclerosis (ALS, or Lou Gehrig's disease), Alzheimer's disease, and multiple sclerosis.

OBESITY

Some studies have shown that people who are deficient in vitamin D are more likely to be obese. However, it is difficult to know whether low vitamin D levels cause obesity or obesity causes low vitamin D levels. Low levels of vitamin D also correlate with a higher incidence of type 2 diabetes.

DEFICIENCY AND TOXICITY

Because sunlight is so important for vitamin D production in the body, some populations are especially at risk for vitamin D deficiency. These include people who live in cloudy or cool northern climates, people who don't spend much time outdoors, those who keep most of their skin covered, and people who typically use sunblock.

Exposure to the sun cannot create too much vitamin D in your body, but toxicity can occur through long-term ingestion of daily supplements. Symptoms of excess vitamin D include heart arrhythmia and increased calcium in the blood. The National Institutes of Health suggests that symptoms are unlikely at less than 10,000 IU per day.

RECOMMENDED AMOUNTS AND FOOD SOURCES

When the sun's ultraviolet rays hit your skin, your body absorbs them and synthesizes them into vitamin D. This is your body's primary source of vitamin D. If you can, spend 10 to 15 minutes in the sun each day with your skin exposed. You can also get vitamin D from dietary sources, including fatty fish like salmon and tuna. Mushrooms also contain vitamin D, as do egg yolks and cheese. In the United States, you can also purchase milk that has been fortified with vitamin D, which also helps your body absorb the calcium that the milk contains. You may find vitamin D in other fortified foods, such as cereal, orange juice, and milk alternatives like soymilk and almond milk. If you are concerned about vitamin D deficiencies due to the relatively small amounts contained in foods, talk with your health care practitioner about supplementation.

vitamins

RDA: VITAMIN D

The National Institutes of Health dietary recommendations for vitamin D are as follows:

0 to 12 months	400 IU
1 to 70 years	600 IU
71 years and older	800 IU
Pregnant and lactating females	600 IU

VITAMIN E SUPPLEMENTS

Vitamin E supplementation may be problematic. Recent research suggests that vitamin E supplementation may actually increase the risk of developing certain types of cancer and heart disease. Therefore, it's best to avoid supplementation, or at least discuss it with your doctor before making a decision. That doesn't mean, however, that eating foods rich in vitamin E is harmful to your health. It is, in fact, beneficial. The issues occur only with supplementation.

VITAMIN E

Vitamin E is a fat-soluble vitamin. This vitamin exists in eight forms: alpha-, beta-, delta-, and gamma-tocopherol, and alpha-, beta-, delta-, and gamma-tocotrienol. The form your body uses the most is alpha-tocopherol.

ANTIOXIDANT

Vitamin E works in the body as an antioxidant. It helps fight or reverse damage caused by free radicals in the body, which are the result of oxidative stress or damaging practices such as smoking. Therefore, it may play a role in the prevention or progression of disease.

CANCER

Studies show a correlation between high dietary levels of vitamin E and a reduced rate of development of cancer, which suggests that consuming vitamin E–rich foods may have a protective effect. However, no correlation has been shown between vitamin E supplementation and a reduced risk of cancer.

CIRCULATORY SYSTEM

Vitamin E helps the body synthesize vitamin K, which is essential for blood clotting. It also aids in the production of red blood cells and widens blood vessels, which can help prevent blockages and the development of clots.

HEART DISEASE

Along with preventing clot formation, vitamin E may be important in preventing heart disease via other mechanisms. Population studies show that higher levels of vitamin E correlate with a reduced risk of heart disease; however, specific studies haven't validated a causal link between the two.

IMMUNITY

Vitamin E plays a key role in the body's immune system. It helps keep the immune response strong, allowing you to fight off minor and major diseases. This vitamin is especially important for older people.

VISION

There is some evidence that vitamin E and other antioxidants provide protection against age-related macular degeneration, and vitamin E combined with vitamin C may treat an inflammatory condition of the eye called uveitis.

DEFICIENCY AND TOXICITY

Vitamin E deficiency may arise in people who consume inadequate amounts, or in those with fat malabsorption issues such as lack of a gallbladder. Deficiencies may cause a number of symptoms including weakness, muscle loss, vision problems, or liver and kidney problems.

Because vitamin E is a fat-soluble vitamin, supplementation can cause it to build up to toxic levels. One study showed that supplementation of vitamin E actually increased the risk of stroke, although the results remain controversial. Another showed that men supplementing vitamin E had a higher risk of developing prostate cancer, while yet another showed it reduced the risk. What these results may suggest is that supplementation isn't the best way to get your vitamin E. Instead, try eating foods rich in vitamin E, which will not cause toxicity. If you do feel you need to supplement, talk with your doctor first.

Symptoms associated with vitamin E toxicity include increased risk of bleeding and brain hemorrhage. If you do take supplemental vitamin E, you should not take it if you are taking blood thinners, because the combination can increase these risks.

RECOMMENDED AMOUNTS AND FOOD SOURCES

Vitamin E is present in a number of dietary sources, including eggs, tree nuts, sunflower seeds, dark leafy greens, avocados, sweet potatoes, and liver. Because there does seem to be some risk involved in taking supplemental vitamin E, your best bet is to obtain this essential nutrient from food sources, which don't present the same risks.

vitamins

RDA: VITAMIN E

Dietary recommendations from the National Institutes of Health's Office of Dietary Supplements are as follows:

0 to 6 months	4 mg (6 IU)
7 to 12 months	5 mg (7.5 IU)
1 to 3 years	6 mg (9 IU)
4 to 8 years	7 mg (10.4 IU)
9 to 13 years	11 mg (16.4 IU)
14 years and older	15 mg (22.4 IU)
Pregnant females	15 mg (22.4 IU)
Lactating females	19 mg (28.4 IU)

VITAMIN OVERDOSE

It's nearly impossible to overdose on water-soluble vitamins, because your body just uses what it needs and excretes any excess amounts in your urine. The vitamins most at risk for overdose or toxicity are vitamins E and A. Therefore, these are best obtained from food sources and not from supplements.

MULTIVITAMIN SUPPLEMENTS

If you're eating a varied diet that is high in colorful plants and contains moderate amounts of animal foods, chances are you're getting the nutrients you need; this is even more likely if your diet consists mostly of unprocessed, whole foods. However, if you eat the Standard American Diet—high in empty calories and processed foods— chances are that a good-quality multivitamin supplement might be a sensible choice.

VITAMIN K

Vitamin K is a fat-soluble vitamin that is necessary for blood clotting. Infants are born without vitamin K, which is why hospitals routinely administer a vitamin K shot at birth.

BLOOD CLOTTING

According to the Harvard T. H. Chan School of Public Health, vitamin K makes four of the thirteen proteins necessary for blood to clot. It is also necessary for the formation of several other clotting factors, so it is very important in preventing hemorrhage. People who take blood thinners need to make sure they also consume adequate levels of vitamin K in order to prevent excessive bleeding.

BONE HEALTH

Vitamin K also increases the mineral density of bones, keeping them strong. It does this by helping your body use calcium to build and mineralize bones. Some studies show that supplementing vitamin K or consuming adequate levels of it may reduce the rate of fractures in people with osteoporosis. This occurs because vitamin K works in synergy with vitamin D to improve bone density and mineralization.

CANCER

Vitamin K hasn't been widely studied in relation to cancer prevention. One researcher at the Office of Cancer Complementary and Alternative Medicine at the National Cancer Institute is studying vitamin K_1 for prevention and treatment of liver cancer, but results haven't provided much evidence for or against its use at this time.

HEART DISEASE

Recent research suggests that vitamin K may help minimize calcification in arteries, a process which can lead to heart attack and heart disease. One form, menaquinone (vitamin K_2), may provide more protective benefits against arterial calcification than the other form, phylloquinone (vitamin K_1). Results from this research are preliminary, and more studies are needed to isolate the effects of vitamin K_2 on arterial calcification, but initial results remain promising. If you have heart disease, talk to your doctor about using vitamin K_2 in this capacity.

DEFICIENCY AND TOXICITY

Vitamin K deficiency may occur in people with fat malabsorption issues, as well as those with an unhealthy diet. Deficiency of this vitamin increases the risk of hemorrhage or poor blood clotting.

Although it is a fat-soluble vitamin, natural vitamin K does not appear to be toxic even at high levels. If you are concerned about toxicity, consume your vitamin K from foods and not from supplements.

RECOMMENDED AMOUNTS AND FOOD SOURCES

Eating dark leafy greens will provide very high levels of vitamin K. Other foods high in this nutrient include parsley, broccoli, Brussels sprouts, cabbage, celery, green beans, summer squash, winter squash, and raspberries. If you eat a varied diet with plenty of colorful plant foods, you will get all the vitamin K your body requires.

RDA: VITAMIN K

Recommendations from the IOM are as follows:

0 to 6 months	2 mcg (AI)
7 to 12 months	2.5 mcg (AI)
1 to 3 years	30 mcg
4 to 8 years	55 mcg
9 to 13 years	60 mcg
14 to 18 years	75 mcg
Males 19 years and older	120 mcg
Females 19 years and older	90 mcg
Pregnant and lactating females up to 18 years	75 mcg
Pregnant and lactating females 19 years and older	90 mcg

Minerals are chemical elements that appear in trace amounts in food. Your body requires some minerals to function, while others may be harmful in large amounts.

minerals

ALUMINUM

Aluminum is the most abundant metallic element on earth, making up about 12 percent of the earth's crust. This mineral is found in every biological entity on the planet—animal, plant, and human. Aluminum is not considered highly toxic because it is not easily available. However, it is not considered nutritionally beneficial for living organisms, either. Aluminum can interfere with the absorption of calcium, iron, and magnesium because it has a similar size and electrical charge to these minerals. When someone is healthy, only about 0.3 percent of ingested aluminum is absorbed and then eliminated through the kidneys. Anyone with impaired kidney function, especially those on dialysis, can have an elevated concentration of aluminum. Eating acidic foods that have been cooked in or served in an aluminum container can significantly boost the absorption rate of the mineral, too. The amount of aluminum found in the human body is about 65 mg. When the quantity of absorbed aluminum is higher than the body's capacity to get rid of it, the excess mineral is stored in tissues such as muscle, lung, kidneys, thyroid, brain, heart, bone, liver, and spleen.

ALZHEIMER'S DISEASE

One concern about aluminum that sparked a media storm is its perceived link to Alzheimer's disease. High levels of aluminum in the brain tissue of people suffering from Alzheimer's invited theories about aluminum's possible role, but there are also studies that refute a link. A 1992 study found identical levels of aluminum in Alzheimer's patients and in the non-Alzheimer's control group. These findings create real doubt about whether aluminum is actually linked to the disease.

DEFICIENCY AND TOXICITY

There is no concern about an aluminum deficiency, because the mineral has no known essential function in the body. However, an excess of aluminum can manifest in a variety of symptoms. Even slightly elevated levels of aluminum can create subtle indicators:

* An aversion to meat
* Stunted growth in infants
* Anorexia
* Colic
* Constipation
* Dry mucous membranes
* Dry skin
* Flatulence
* Headaches
* Heartburn
* Lack of energy
* Muscle twitching
* Repeated colds
* Skin rashes

If exposure continues and the body does not eliminate the aluminum, serious symptoms and diseases could develop. These conditions are not definitively linked to aluminum, but some studies seem to point in that direction. Other symptoms and diseases associated with long-term aluminum toxicity are as follows:

* Alzheimer's disease
* Anemia
* Colitis
* Hemolysis
* Hypoparathyroidism
* Kidney dysfunction
* Liver dysfunction
* Loss of memory
* Neuromuscular disorders
* Paralytic muscular conditions
* Parkinson's disease
* Ulcers

Aluminum toxicity should be treated to avoid severe symptoms. The first step is to limit exposure to aluminum and allow the body to eliminate what is present without further accumulation. A chelating agent such as tetracycline (taken orally) or ethylenediaminetetraacetic acid (EDTA) administered through an IV can clear aluminum from the body more rapidly. The most effective method to determine levels of aluminum in the body is a hair analysis accompanied by urine and blood tests. A normal hair reading for aluminum is under 10 to 15 ppm.

RECOMMENDED AMOUNTS AND FOOD SOURCES

There is no known benefit of aluminum in the body, but there are trace amounts of aluminum in everything you eat or drink, and diet is the main source of exposure. Natural sources of aluminum include tea (which contains very high concentrations), most fruits and vegetables, beer, wine, beef, eggs, coffee, fish, ham, and poultry. Nonfood sources of aluminum include antacids, the coating on aspirin, ground and tap water, cosmetics, cookware, and aluminum foil. The average intake from natural sources is 2 to 10 mg per day and total absorption of about 10 to 110 mg.

BISMUTH

Bismuth is a heavy metal but not considered to be as toxic as lead or arsenic. It is about 86 percent as dense as lead, and some countries, such as Denmark, the United States, and England, use it as a replacement for the more toxic metal for plumbing and soldering purposes. Bismuth may be better known in the United States as part of the compound that makes up Pepto-Bismol (bismuth subsalicylate), but it is also used for other purposes:

* Coloring agent in cosmetics
* Treatment for eye infections
* Ingredient in burn ointments
* Fungicide
* Treatment for warts
* Treatment for syphilis
* Aid in reducing the odor of excrement in colostomy patients

GASTROINTESTINAL DISORDERS

There are not many studies that illustrate possible nutritional impacts from bismuth, but this metal is extremely absorbent, which can reduce the acidity of the stomach and remove toxins from the intestines. These properties make bismuth or compounds such as bismuth subsalicylate an extremely effective ingredient in treatments for peptic ulcers, heartburn, nausea, diarrhea, and gastrointestinal diseases. The development of peptic ulcers used to be blamed on stress and other lifestyle choices, but the true culprit responsible for this health issue is a bacterium called *Helicobacter pylori,* which causes a gastric infection. Bismuth compounds were used extensively as a treatment for these ulcers because medical professionals assumed that bismuth acted as a barrier to stomach acid. It was not known initially that the treatment was effective because *H. pylori* is vulnerable to the antimicrobial activity of bismuth.

DEFICIENCY AND TOXICITY

There are no issues associated with a bismuth deficiency because it is not considered to be essential to human health. With normal exposure, the daily intake of bismuth is less than 5 mcg per day, and the body effectively excretes it. When ingested, bismuth is excreted through feces, and when absorbed it mainly leaves the body in urine. Despite an impressive excretion rate, bismuth can still be found in small quantities in human tissues, but this might be due to environmental exposure and use of cosmetics or medications that contain bismuth. Concentrations of this element are highest in the kidneys, lungs, liver, and lymph nodes. These levels are not usually damaging, but accumulation can occur if exposure is high.

Bismuth toxicity can occur through excessive exposure to antacids, anti-diarrheal medications, ulcer medications, some drinking water, cosmetics, pigments and paints, and batteries, and in professions such as metal mining and refining. High levels of bismuth can inactivate enzymes, affect the mucous membranes, and have a negative impact on the brain and nerves. Symptoms include a dark-colored tongue, respiratory issues, confusion, depression, weakness, decreased appetite, dark-colored gums, joint pain, skin rash, tremors, muscle spasms, diarrhea, and black stools.

MENOPAUSE

After menopause, women may have different nutritional needs. Because the metabolism slows down, you may require fewer calories to maintain your current weight than you once did. If you were supplementing iron before menopause due to anemia, there's a good chance you won't need to do so any longer. It is important to talk to your doctor about discontinuing the supplementation. Likewise, you may require more calcium and vitamin D to prevent osteoporosis, and to lower salt intake in order to control your blood pressure.

RECOMMENDED AMOUNTS AND FOOD SOURCES

There are not many dietary sources of bismuth, but the metal can be found in some sea vegetables, roots, and tubers such as kelp and maca root. You will not find it as a supplement, either. Bismuth is a common ingredient in cosmetics and in medications such as Pepto-Bismol and Kaopectate. These types of gastrointestinal treatment medications are the main source of bismuth for most people. Again, when used in excessive amounts, bismuth compounds can lead to side effects, so it is important to consult with a medical professional before using it. There is no RDA for bismuth because it is not considered to be essential to human health.

CALCIUM

Calcium is the most plentiful mineral in the human body and is best known as a component of bones and teeth. Indeed, about 99 percent of the calcium in the body is stored in the bones and teeth, where it can be used onsite or enter the bloodstream to be used in other metabolic functions. Bones are constantly reconstructing, which means that calcium is being reabsorbed and deposited to create new bone. When the balance shifts from formation to bone breakdown, there is an increased risk of osteoporosis. The remaining 1 percent of calcium stored in the body is used for muscle contraction, including vascular contraction and vasodilation, intracellular signaling, blood clotting, nerve transmission, hormone secretion, and cellular metabolism.

The absorption rate of calcium is about 30 percent, but infants and children absorb more, and the rate decreases as people get older. Eating foods high in oxalic acid and phytic acid can reduce the absorption rate of calcium, and vitamin D is required for calcium to move from the digestive tract. Absorbed calcium is eliminated in sweat, urine, and feces. The amount that is lost depends on several factors:

* High sodium levels, which can increase the excretion rate
* Caffeine, which can decrease absorption and increase excretion
* Alcohol, which can reduce the absorption rate and prevent vitamin D from converting to an active form

* High fruit and vegetable intake, which can create an alkaline environment in the body, thereby decreasing calcium absorption

DEFICIENCY AND TOXICITY

Calcium deficiency usually does not produce any significant symptoms in the short term, but long-term effects can be damaging. Hypocalcemia, a condition marked by chronically low calcium levels, increases the risk of bone fractures and eventually leads to osteoporosis. People with a higher risk of calcium deficiency include postmenopausal women, those who are lactose intolerant, vegetarians, and amenorrheic women. Hypocalcemia symptoms can include muscle cramps, memory loss, brittle nails, dermatitis, irregular heartbeat, poor appetite, mental confusion, skeletal malformations, numbness or tingling in the extremities, hallucinations, depression, convulsions, fatigue, and, if left untreated, death.

Moderately high levels of calcium, usually from supplements, can cause constipation and interfere with the absorption of minerals such as zinc and iron. Excessive calcium has also been linked to a higher risk of kidney stones, prostate cancer, and cardiovascular disease, although more research is required to solidify those connections. Extremely high levels of calcium in the blood can produce a condition called hypercalcemia, which can cause vascular calcification, hypercaliuria (excessive calcium in the urine), and renal insufficiency.

RECOMMENDED AMOUNTS AND FOOD SOURCES

Most people in the United States get about half of their calcium from dairy products, but there are many other good dietary sources of calcium, such as sardines, dark leafy greens, almonds, broccoli, fortified cereals, white beans, soybeans, bok choy, black-eyed peas, oranges, sesame seeds, okra, green beans, fortified orange juice, dried figs, rhubarb, and salmon. You can also get calcium from supplements in two forms, carbonate and citrate.

Children need a large quantity of calcium for new bone growth, and older individuals need extra to offset a lower absorption rate after 40 years of age. People in the United States, especially women, often fall short of adequate amounts of calcium.

minerals

RDA: CALCIUM

The RDA of calcium is not the amount needed to prevent a deficiency, but rather the amount needed to offset net calcium loss:

0 to 6 months	200 mg (AI)
7 to 12 months	260 mg (AI)
1 to 3 years	700 mg
4 to 8 years	1,000 mg
9 to 18 years	1,300 mg
19 to 50 years	1,000 mg
Males 50 to 71 years	1,000 mg
Females 51 to 70 years	1,200 mg
71 years and older	1,200 mg
Pregnant and lactating females up to 18 years	1,300 mg
Pregnant and lactating females 19 years and up	1,000 mg

CHLORIDE

Chloride is a mineral that is essential for good health. It is an electrolyte as well, which means it is water-soluble and carries an electrical charge—a negative one in chloride's case. This electrical charge allows chloride to move freely across cell membranes so it can carry in other nutrients and carry out waste and water. Chloride is easily absorbed and excreted by the body. In conjunction with water, potassium, and sodium, chloride helps regulate the distribution of fluids in the body. Chloride is absorbed by the body in the intestines and then excreted through sweat, vomit, and urine. The kidneys will excrete or hold on to chloride in order to balance the pH in the body. This mineral is predominantly found in gastrointestinal secretions and cerebrospinal fluid, as well as in plasma and interstitial fluid, where it is crucial for the electrolyte and fluid balance that helps maintain healthy blood pressure and blood volume.

Chloride is also an important component of gastric juice because it forms hydrochloric acid when combined with hydrogen molecules. This acid breaks down the food you eat into smaller particles in the stomach so that the small intestine can easily absorb them. A normal acidic environment created by adequate chloride levels in the body is important for the absorption of nutrients such as protein, vitamin B_{12}, and iron.

DEFICIENCY AND TOXICITY

A deficiency of chloride, or hypochloremia, can occur due to excessive vomiting, diarrhea, heavy use of laxatives or diuretics, some kidney disorders, and Addison's disease. It can also occur when infants are fed chloride-deficient formula. When chloride levels drop too low, a life-threatening condition called alkalosis can occur. Alkalosis means that the blood pH is too alkaline, and its symptoms can include lethargy, muscle fatigue, irritability, dehydration, and loss of appetite.

An excess of chloride, known as hyperchloremia, is theoretically possible, especially in those who consume a diet high in processed foods. Levels of chloride in the body often mirror sodium levels, because of the prevalence of salt in most standard diets. High levels of chloride and sodium together create water retention, high blood pressure, and an increased risk of atherosclerosis. Other than high salt intake, hyperchloremia can also be caused by dehydration; reduced urine output due to kidney disease, cancer, or gastritis; a bladder stone; and some medications. You are more likely to have a chloride deficiency than an excess of this mineral in your body. The body excretes chlorine rapidly through urine and sweat, so hot weather and exertion that produces excessive perspiration can create a chloride deficiency.

RECOMMENDED AMOUNTS AND FOOD SOURCES

Chloride is present in many foods, and getting an adequate amount through diet should be easily achievable. Most people get the majority of their chloride as sodium chloride in salt. This is not the best source of this essential nutrient, but salt intake can help keep chloride levels in a healthy range for effective body function. It is important to monitor salt intake if that is your main source of chloride, because too much salt can create many health issues. Other sources of chloride include kelp, olives, rye, cocoa, tomatoes, lettuce, cheese, legumes, whole grains, and celery.

CHROMIUM

Chromium is considered to be a trace mineral, and more research is required to determine exactly how much is needed for optimal health. The absorption rate of chromium in the small intestine is not high, about 0.4 to 2.5 percent, and the unabsorbed mineral is excreted through feces. The liver, soft tissues, spleen, and bones contain most of the body's stored chromium. You can increase the absorption rate of chromium by including vitamin C and niacin in your meals. Factors that reduce the rate of absorption are a diet high in simple sugars, pregnancy and lactation, intense exercise, stress, and infection.

Chromium can improve the action of insulin and plays a role in the metabolism of carbohydrates, fats, and proteins in the body, which can help stabilize blood sugar. This means that chromium might be an effective treatment to control diabetes and support weight loss. Studies have shown that chromium supplements (between 200 mcg and 400 mcg) can normalize blood sugar levels, decrease insulin requirements in people who are insulin resistant, reduce triglycerides and LDL cholesterol, reduce carbohydrate cravings, and reduce fat mass.

minerals

RDA: CHLORIDE

The currently established RDA is as follows:

0 to 6 months	180 mg
7 to 12 months	570 mg
1 to 3 years	1,500 mg
4 to 8 years	1,900 mg
9 to 50 years	2,300 mg
51 to 70 years	2,000 mg
71 years and older	1,800 mg
Pregnant and lactating females	2,300 mg

SUPERFOOD: AÇAÍ

A few years ago, some unscrupulous companies were selling açaí supplements as a fast way to lose weight. While these marketing campaigns were patently false, they don't negate the powerful health benefits of the açaí berry. Açaí is high in antioxidants, particularly anthocyanins. It is also high in omega-3 fatty acids and oleic acid (which is also present in olive oil). You can probably find flash-frozen açaí berries at your supermarket, and they are wonderful when added to smoothies. Avoid açaí juice, which tends to be relatively high in sugar content.

DEFICIENCY AND TOXICITY

Chromium deficiency is not a common issue but can occur when people are on intravenous feeding without added chromium, or if their diet is very poor. Chromium is very important for the metabolism of carbohydrates, so many of the symptoms associated with a deficiency seem connected to blood sugar. Mild deficiency of chromium can manifest as fatigue, nervousness, and unstable blood sugar levels. More serious chromium deficiency symptoms can include:

* Anxiety
* Blurred vision
* Confusion
* Depression
* Dizziness
* Elevated blood cholesterol
* Elevated blood triglycerides
* Excessive thirst
* Hunger
* Hyperactivity
* Hypocholesterolemia
* Lack of energy
* Mood swings
* Negative nitrogen balance
* Prediabetes
* Sweating

Chromium is not absorbed well, so unless you are supplementing this mineral in large amounts it is unlikely that an excess will occur in your body from dietary sources. Severe chromium exposure in an environmental or occupational setting is possible and usually occurs through inhalation of chromium dust or through skin contact. Symptoms can include:

* Gastrointestinal irritation (nausea, vomiting, and diarrhea)
* Vertigo
* Asthma
* Chronic bronchitis

- * Chronic pharyngitis
- * Chronic rhinitis
- * Congestion
- * Polyps in the upper respiratory tract
- * Erythema
- * Fissuring of the skin
- * Papules
- * Skin scaling
- * Swelling
- * Muscle cramps
- * Toxic nephritis
- * Renal failure
- * Circulatory collapse
- * Liver damage
- * Acute multisystem organ failure
- * Coma

These symptoms can result from either an acute or long-term exposure to chromium dust or skin contact, not from diet. Those who work in chromite industries also have a higher risk of developing lung, sinus, and nasal cancer.

RECOMMENDED AMOUNTS AND FOOD SOURCES
Chromium is found in meats, seafood, poultry, dairy, grains, legumes, seeds, vegetables, and fruits, but many foods contain only a tiny amount of this mineral, less than 2 mcg. The amount of chromium in foods can fluctuate depending on the type of agriculture that produces it and whether the food is processed. Good sources of chromium include broccoli, mussels, Brazil nuts, barley, oats, brewer's yeast, green beans, oysters, dates, pears, tomatoes, romaine lettuce, black pepper, apples, milk, corn, sweet potatoes, and mushrooms.

In the United States, most men consume 39 to 54 mcg of chromium per day, which is more than adequate, and women consume 23 to 29 mcg per day, which is adequate unless they are pregnant or breast-feeding.

RDA: CHROMIUM

The National Academy of Sciences recommends the following adequate intake levels per day for chromium:

0 to 6 months	0.2 mcg
7 to 12 months	5.5 mcg
1 to 3 years	11 mcg
4 to 8 years	15 mcg
Males 9 to 13 years	25 mcg
Males 14 to 50 years	35 mcg
Males 51 years and older	30 mcg
Females 9 to 13 years	21 mcg
Females 14 to 18 years	24 mcg
Females 19 to 50 years	25 mcg
Females 51 years and older	20 mcg
Pregnant females	30 mcg
Lactating females	45 mcg

COPPER

Copper is an essential trace element that is critical for many body functions. Very little copper is stored in the body, about 80 to 100 mg, or less than the amount in a penny. Copper is stored mostly in the liver, brain, and muscles. When copper is ingested, about 30 percent is rapidly absorbed in the stomach and small intestine. After being transferred across the gut wall by water-soluble proteins, copper travels to the liver, where it becomes a copper-protein complex called ceruloplasmin. Ceruloplasmin represents about 90 percent of the copper in the blood and is crucial for iron storage and transportation. Copper is a cofactor (a necessary part of the process) of many enzymes that impact numerous important functions:

* Strengthening of collagen in blood vessels, cartilage, tendons, and bones
* Synthesis of a neurotransmitter and adrenal hormone called norepinephrine
* Energy production from the transfer of electrons caused by the oxidation of fat, protein, and carbohydrates
* Integration of iron into red blood cells
* Prevention of emphysema and maintenance of healthy lung tissue
* Insulation of nerve cells
* Prevention of oxidative damage

DEFICIENCY AND TOXICITY

A surprising number of people in the United States, between 25 and 50 percent, fall short of the recommended amount of copper each day. The risk of copper deficiency has risen sharply in the last half century due to modern food-processing techniques and copper-depleted soil from commercial farming. Chronic low levels of copper deficiency can create the following symptoms:

* Bone fractures
* Depressed immune system
* Dermatitis
* Diarrhea

- Edema
- Fatigue
- Hair loss
- Impaired glucose tolerance
- Increased cholesterol
- Irregular heartbeat
- Labored respiration
- Low body temperature
- Low white blood cell count
- Oxidative damage
- Poor nerve conductivity

Chronic copper deficiency can lead to an increased risk of cardiovascular disease, thrombosis, osteoporosis, anemia, thyroid issues, osteoarthritis, rheumatoid arthritis, colon cancer, and impaired cognitive function. Some nondietary factors can create a copper deficiency, such as untreated celiac disease, pancreatic cancer, and excessive zinc intake. A rare inherited copper deficiency, Menkes syndrome, can also produce seriously low levels of copper and can be fatal.

Copper toxicity is rare but can occur. One reason for excessive copper levels is drinking water that runs through copper pipes. Copper can leach into the water running through the pipes, especially if the water sits in the pipes and is hot. If you have a metallic taste in your water or your sinks and faucets have greenish staining, get the copper levels tested. Running cold water through the pipes for several minutes before using the water and cooking with cold water can reduce the copper levels. Symptoms of excess copper can include nausea, vomiting, headache, diarrhea, weakness, dizziness; more severe copper toxicity can cause cardiovascular issues, liver problems, coma, and even death.

The second most common reason for copper toxicity is a rare inherited condition called Wilson's disease, which causes a buildup of copper in the liver, kidneys, brain, and eyes. People with Wilson's disease cannot clear excess copper from their body, and this gives rise to problems such as fatigue, jaundice, trouble swallowing, muscle stiffness, abdominal pain,

minerals

RDA: COPPER

The recommended daily dietary intake of copper from the IOM is as follows:

0 to months	200 mcg
7 to 12 months	220 mcg
1 to 3 years	340 mcg
4 to 8 years	440 mcg
9 to 13 years	700 mcg
14 to 18 years	890 mcg
19 years and older	900 mcg
Pregnant females	1,000 mcg (1 mg)
Lactating females	1,300 mcg (1.3 mg)

fluid buildup in the legs, and issues with coordination. Wilson's disease is treatable with a low copper diet and medication.

RECOMMENDED AMOUNTS AND FOOD SOURCES

Most foods have tiny amounts of copper, and the best sources are whole, unprocessed foods. Dietary sources of copper include seafood, organ meats, nuts, seeds, legumes, chocolate, whole grains, black pepper, blackstrap molasses, dark leafy greens, avocados, asparagus, mushrooms, squash, tomatoes, potatoes, sweet potatoes, bananas, grapes, olives, pineapple, beets, raspberries, and tomatoes.

minerals

FLUORIDE

Fluoride is a trace element that is important for dental health. There are approximately 2.6 g of fluoride present in adults, about 99 percent of which is located in the bones and teeth. When ingested, fluoride is absorbed in the stomach and small intestine into the bloodstream, where it travels to mineralized tissue such as teeth and bones. Adults store about 60 percent of the fluoride ingested, and infants store between 80 and 90 percent. Excess fluoride is excreted in the urine.

The primary use of fluoride in the body is preventing tooth decay. Fluoride increases bone stability and hardens the enamel on teeth. Information compiled from studies between 1976 and 1987 shows that adding fluoride to drinking water reduces the incidence of dental caries by 30 to 60 percent in children and up to 35 percent in adults. Children who ingested fluoride before their adult teeth erupted had an increased resistance to cavities in adulthood. Fluoride is also used as a treatment for osteoporosis because it increases bone mass. This increased mass does not seem to decrease the risk of fractures, so more testing is required to determine the benefits of fluoride.

DEFICIENCY AND TOXICITY

Insufficient fluoride intake can cause an increased risk of tooth decay. Before the introduction of fluoride to toothpastes, areas with the recommended fluoride concentrations in the water showed markedly lower incidence of dental caries, by about 40 to 60 percent. Chronic long-term fluoride deficiency has also been linked to osteoporosis.

Excess fluoride before the eruption of adult teeth can cause dental fluorosis, which manifests as spots or white flecks on the teeth, or mottling and staining in more serious cases. Excess fluoride can be toxic if ingested in large quantities, causing these symptoms:

* Weakness
* Tremors
* Convulsions
* A salty taste in the mouth
* Excessive saliva
* Nausea
* Cramps and diarrhea
* Vomiting
* Sweating
* Calcium deficiency
* Death (in extreme cases)

The more extreme symptoms are usually caused by fluoride used as a treatment for osteoporosis. These patients need to ensure their calcium intake is sufficient and to closely monitor their physical state. High fluoride intake also causes a condition called skeletal fluorosis, characterized by increased bone mass, stiffness, and joint pain.

RECOMMENDED AMOUNTS AND FOOD SOURCES

Fluoridated tap water is the most significant source of fluoride for people in the United States. About 0.7 mg of fluoride per liter of water is added to drinking water in most municipalities to help prevent dental caries. Most foods also contain trace amounts of fluoride, but tea, fish, and infant formulas contain high fluoride levels. Some fruits contain higher amounts, due to the application of superphosphate fertilizers, which contain fluorides. The addition of water containing fluoride to food such as baby formulas, and cooking foods in fluoridated water, can increase the levels of this mineral in the food. Children often increase their intake of fluoride when they swallow fluoride toothpaste.

RDA: FLUORIDE

The data required to determine an RDA for fluoride is insufficient, so the IOM created an adequate intake level based on the amount of fluoride needed to reduce dental caries safely:

0 to 6 months	0.01 mg
7 to 12 months	0.5 mg
1 to 3 years	0.7 mg
4 to 8 years	1 mg
9 to 13 years	2 mg
14 to 18 years	3 mg
Males 19 years and older	4 mg
Females 19 years and older	3 mg
Pregnant and lactating females	3 mg

IODINE

Iodine is a trace element that is essential to healthy thyroid function. A common dietary form of iodine is iodide, a salt that is absorbed very quickly in the stomach and small intestine. Iodide then travels to the thyroid gland, where it is used in thyroid hormone synthesis, and any excess is excreted in the urine. Most adults store 15 to 20 mg of iodine, 70 to 80 percent of which is in the thyroid gland. Iodine is a component of the thyroid hormones triiodothyronine (T_3) and thyroxine (T_4). Thyroid function is controlled by thyroid stimulating hormone (TSH), which is secreted by the pituitary gland. TSH protects the body from hypothyroidism and hyperthyroidism by increasing the uptake of iodine into the thyroid and promoting the production and release of T_3 and T_4. Thyroid hormones are responsible for many reactions in the body, including enzyme activity, protein synthesis, and metabolism, as well as healthy nervous system and skeletal development in fetuses and children.

DEFICIENCY AND TOXICITY

Iodine deficiency used to be a serious issue, especially in areas with iodine-deficient soil and limited access to seafood on a regular basis. Iodized salt lessened this issue considerably, but certain parts of the world are still vulnerable, such as mountainous regions as well as Southeast Asia. In addition, some foods, such as soy, cruciferous vegetables, and cassava, contain substances called goitrogens, which can interfere with the absorption of iodine. A diet high in these foods can contribute to iodine deficiency. Iodine deficiency (hypothyroidism) in adults occurs when dietary intake is less than 10 to 20 mcg per day and produces a goiter, or visibly enlarged thyroid. Since thyroid hormones are also used by many other tissues, an iodine deficiency can affect those areas negatively as well. Hypothyroidism can produce dry mouth, dry skin, scar tissue, fibrosis, mental fogginess, fibromyalgia, hair loss, and impaired saliva production.

Iodine deficiency is especially damaging during pregnancy and childhood. Even mildly to moderately low iodine levels can affect the development of the fetus and impair cognitive function in children. Symptoms of mild iodine deficiency during this stage of development include lower-than-average intelligence and an increased risk for ADHD. Severe iodine deficiency can produce mental retardation, stunted growth, deafness, motor function issues, and delayed maturation, as well as miscarriage and stillbirth.

The symptoms of excess iodine in adults can be the same as for deficiency—hypothyroidism and goiter. Hyperthyroidism is usually the result of treatment for an iodine deficiency. Chronic doses of iodine in excessive amounts can cause thyroid papillary cancer and thyroiditis. Acute iodine poisoning is very rare; the symptoms include fever, burning of the digestive tract, nausea, cramps, weak pulse, and coma.

RECOMMENDED AMOUNTS AND FOOD SOURCES

Iodine naturally occurs in food, but the amount can fluctuate depending on the concentration of iodine in the soil and farming techniques. The foods that are considered to be good sources of iodine are seaweed, seafood, whole grains, dairy products, eggs, fruits, and vegetables. Iodized salt is also a common source of iodine in most countries. In the more than 70 countries that have added iodine to salt for decades, iodine deficiencies have dropped considerably. Iodine is also available in multivitamins as potassium iodide or sodium iodide.

The average intake of iodine per day in the United States is adequate, between 138 and 353 mcg. Intake can be in the low range because many people are dependent on processed foods, and the salt added to these products is not usually iodized. People who do not eat seafood can also have low iodine levels.

IRON

Iron is an essential mineral that is needed for the production of red blood cells. It is a component of the protein hemoglobin. Hemoglobin transfers oxygen from the lungs to the tissues, and the protein myoglobin in turn provides oxygen to the muscles. Iron is also crucial for cell function, synthesis of enzymes, brain development, the conversion of blood sugar to energy, and growth.

minerals

RDA: IODINE

The RDA for iodine is as follows:

0 to 6 months	110 mcg
7 to 12 months	130 mcg
1 to 8 years	90 mcg
9 to 13 years	120 mcg
14 years and older	150 mcg
Pregnant females	220 mcg
Lactating females	290 mcg

Iron is absorbed from the stomach and duodenum and carried by transferrin, a protein, to bone marrow, tissues, and organs. A copper-containing protein called ceruloplasmin is also required to transport iron to the brain. Approximately 4 grams of iron are found in the hemoglobin; the rest is stored in a protein called ferritin. The brain contains large amounts of ferritin, as do muscle tissue, bone marrow, the liver, and the spleen. About 90 percent of dietary iron is unabsorbed and ends up in cells called enterocytes, which are excreted in feces.

Dietary iron can either be in heme or nonheme form. Heme iron is typically found in animal proteins, while nonheme iron most commonly occurs in plants and fortified foods. Heme iron is absorbed better than nonheme iron. The absorption rates of iron can be also affected by other factors that affect the bioavailability of the iron in the food source:

* Eating heme-iron sources with nonheme-iron foods can increase the nonheme absorption rate.
* Foods containing phytates, calcium, and polyphenols, such as spinach, tea, dairy, legumes, and whole grains, can decrease nonheme iron absorption.
* Foods containing vitamin C can increase nonheme iron absorption.
* Antacids can reduce iron absorption.

DEFICIENCY AND TOXICITY

Iron deficiency is the most common nutritional issue in the United States, and women have a greater risk of developing this problem. Many physical signs of mild iron deficiency are subtle or nonexistent until symptoms of iron deficiency anemia are evident:

* Anxiety
* Cold extremities
* Cravings for ice or dirt
* Decreased immunity
* Fatigue
* Hair loss
* Headaches
* Inability to concentrate

- ✳ Inflamed tongue
- ✳ Irregular heartbeat
- ✳ Pale gums and skin
- ✳ Restless leg syndrome
- ✳ Shortness of breath

People who may be at a higher risk of iron deficiency include:

- ✳ Pregnant women
- ✳ Infants
- ✳ People with Crohn's disease or celiac disease
- ✳ Frequent blood donors
- ✳ Women with heavy menstruation
- ✳ Vegetarians
- ✳ People diagnosed with cancer
- ✳ People with heart failure
- ✳ Endurance athletes
- ✳ People with anemia or chronic disease

Excessive iron from dietary sources is rare if you are healthy, but taking supplements with high doses of iron can cause constipation, nausea, and, in extreme cases, vomiting, cramps, and faintness. These symptoms are more common if you take iron supplements without food. Extreme iron overdoses can cause convulsions, organ failure, coma, and death. Iron supplements are the most common cause of poisoning in children. An excess buildup of iron can also occur with a disease called hemochromatosis. This disease can be treated with phlebotomy and chelation, but if left untreated, can lead to heart disease, liver cirrhosis, and issues with the pancreas.

RECOMMENDED AMOUNTS AND FOOD SOURCES

Good sources of heme and nonheme iron include shellfish, fish, meat, poultry, legumes, dark leafy greens, fortified cereals, organ meats, soybeans, pumpkin, blackstrap molasses, nuts, eggs, and yeast extract. Iron is also available in dietary supplements including multivitamins and straight iron supplements.

minerals

RDA: IRON

The daily RDA for iron is as follows:

0 to 6 months	0.27 mg (AI)
7 to 12 months	11 mg
1 to 3 years	7 mg
4 to 8 years	10 mg
9 to 13 years	8 mg
Males 14 to 18 years	11 mg
Males 19 and older	8 mg
Females 14 to 18 years	15 mg
Females 19 to 50 years	18 mg
Females 51 years and older	8 mg
Pregnant females	27 mg
Lactating females	10 mg

LEAD

Lead is a toxic mineral. It is the most common contaminant in the human body and environment. Lead naturally occurs deep in the ground, and humans were mostly shielded from dangerous levels of this mineral until the advent of silver smelting, of which lead is a by-product. Early civilizations were exposed to lead through drinking and food containers, as well as through the water pipes in their dwellings. Some researchers believe the downfall of the Roman Empire was hastened due to the ruling class suffering from shortened lifespan and diminished cognitive function from lead toxicity.

Lead is not absorbed easily, and other minerals such as iron and calcium can reduce the absorption rate further. Unfortunately, children have the highest absorption rate. When lead enters the body, most of it is quickly eliminated through the feces and perspiration, making hair analysis the most accurate test for lead poisoning, and urine and blood samples inconclusive. Exposure to this heavy metal is prevalent in North America, where the average estimated body load of lead is 125 to 200 mcg. The United States has many lead-containing products, such as leaded gasoline for older vehicles, paint, food grown near industrial sites or roads, pottery glazes, cosmetic pigments, soldered cans, pesticides, and cigarettes.

Although steps have been taken to reduce lead contamination in the environment (such as the introduction of unleaded gasoline and lead-free paints), people are exposed to lead constantly. With a 5 to 10 percent absorption rate, that exposure quickly adds up to 200 to 400 mcg per day. The body can eliminate this quantity, but clearing rates vary from person to person. The amount of lead considered to be toxic also depends on the individual's age and physical condition. Children and pregnant women are the most vulnerable to lead toxicity.

DEFICIENCY AND TOXICITY

Toxicity, not deficiency, of lead in the body is an issue. When someone has lead toxicity, the lead is most often visible in the bones because it can replace calcium. Lead can impair nerve and brain function because it is a neurotoxin that inactivates the enzymes dependent on copper, calcium, zinc, and iron. This can interfere with red blood cell function, reduce hemoglobin synthesis, and damage or kill the cells of the body. Lead is also an immunosuppressant, increasing the body's vulnerability to bacteria, viruses, free radicals, and other heavy metals.

The early symptoms of lead toxicity are quite subtle. People experience fatigue, nightmares, insomnia, muscle aches, headaches, and constipation, as well as depression, memory loss, irritability, high blood pressure, impaired kidney function, and vertigo as the lead levels increase. Children display hyperactivity, learning disorders, and attention deficit problems with low levels of lead toxicity. With high lead levels the symptoms include nausea, abdominal pain, anemia, vomiting, muscle weakness, confusion, hallucinations, and, in acute cases, death.

Lead poisoning can be treated with an IV containing EDTA, which is a strong chelating agent that latches on to lead and ferries it out in the urine. Administering high levels of calcium will help block lead absorption and improve the excretion rate.

RECOMMENDED AMOUNTS AND FOOD SOURCES

Even though lead is very toxic, studies have shown that it might be beneficial to the body in tiny amounts. The studies concern rats, not humans, but the results merit further testing. Rats consuming small amounts of lead (1 ppm of lead acetate) showed an increased growth rate, about 12 percent over the control group. These test groups exhibited improved hemoglobin and hematocrit concentrations, which suggests that low levels of this mineral might help red blood cell production.

Even so, exposure to lead should be avoided. Lead can enter the body not only through lead-containing products but also through eating plants, which absorb the mineral in the soil. In order to reduce your body lead load, try to eat a nutritionally sound diet packed with minerals and vitamins that will interfere with lead absorption. High fiber and pectin-rich foods will also limit absorption because they help bind all heavy metals, including lead.

SUPERFOOD: CHIA

You've probably heard people touting the benefits of chia, the small seeds that marketers suggest provide endless energy and lots of nutrition. In fact, chia is pretty darn good for you. When you add water and let them sit, chia seeds turn into a gel that may fill you up quickly and keep you from getting hungry between meals. Chia seeds are also a good source of omega-3 fatty acids. They are high in fiber and contain calcium, manganese, magnesium, phosphorus, zinc, vitamins B_1 and B_2, and potassium.

MANGANESE

Manganese is an essential mineral and is crucial for bone growth, healthy nerves, immune system functioning, and blood sugar regulation. Manganese is found in cellular enzymes, in particular in mitochondria. When ingested, the absorption rate of manganese is between 1 and 4 percent, and manganese is then carried to the liver and other tissues to be stored. Most people store 15 to 20 mg in the bones, liver, kidneys, pituitary gland, adrenal glands, and pancreas. Manganese is excreted through feces and bile, with a little in the urine.

This mineral is a cofactor in several enzymes, including manganese superoxide dismutase and prolidase. Manganese superoxide dismutase protects against free radical damage. Prolidase helps make collagen in the skin, which is crucial for wound healing. Manganese also protects the skin from damage as an antioxidant. Manganese helps enzymes convert substances such as amino acids into sugar in a process called gluconeogenesis, which means that manganese plays a role in keeping daily blood sugar levels stable. Manganese is also thought to support bone growth, because a deficiency impairs healthy bone formation.

DEFICIENCY AND TOXICITY

There is not a lot of research on manganese deficiency in people, but some clinical cases are informative. A deficiency in manganese in adults manifests as problems with walking, weakness, weight loss, skin problems, and inner ear noises. A severe deficiency in children may lead to blindness, convulsions, or paralysis. Other foods can inhibit the absorption rate of manganese, such as foods high in phytic acid, tannins, and oxalic acid, and foods very high in iron, phosphorus, and calcium. Low levels of manganese are linked to several chronic diseases such as osteoporosis, diabetes, and epilepsy, although more research is required to determine what role manganese plays in these conditions.

Manganese toxicity from food sources is rare. A high level of manganese in drinking water is associated with neurological symptoms in adults and with behavior problems, hyperactivity, and cognitive deficits in children. Manganese toxicity is found in smelting and welding workers who inhale manganese dust. This dust bypasses the digestive tract and goes directly to the brain. The symptoms of manganese toxicity start with headaches, muscle cramps, fatigue, aggression, and hallucinations, then progress to a condition similar to Parkinson's, with difficulty walking, facial spasms, and tremors.

Some people are more susceptible to excess manganese. Chronic liver disease interferes with manganese excretion because this mineral is eliminated through bile. Children and newborns can also be more vulnerable to manganese toxicity because their absorption rates are higher and excretion rates lower than in adults.

RECOMMENDED AMOUNTS AND FOOD SOURCES

Plant foods are rich in manganese, and the level of manganese in the soil affects the amount present in plants grown in the soil. Commercial farming techniques strip manganese from the soil, resulting in foods with a lower content. The refining process for grains also depletes manganese by about 90 percent. Unprocessed organic foods are the best way to get more manganese in your diet. Most diets provide dietary intakes per day of about 2.3 mg for men and 1.8 mg for women, although vegetarians can reach levels of 10.9 mg. Sources of manganese include whole grains, cinnamon, cloves, strawberries, pineapple, dark leafy greens, legumes, alfalfa, nuts, tea, and coffee.

MAGNESIUM

Magnesium is one of the most crucial elements for human health. Magnesium plays a role in over 300 reactions in the body, and every cell needs this element to function efficiently. The body absorbs between 20 and 50 percent of the magnesium ingested, and there is an amount of about 25 g of magnesium stored in the body, in the bones (about 60 percent), muscles, and soft tissues. Every system in the body is impacted by magnesium. It is needed for:

* Healthy immune system
* Energy metabolism
* Normal blood pressure
* Muscle function

minerals

RDA: MANGANESE

There is no RDA for manganese, but the upper tolerable limit is set at 11 mg per day, which is conservative. An adequate intake level for manganese per day is as follows:

0 to 6 months	0.003 mg
7 to 12 months	0.6 mg
1 to 3 years	1.2 mg
4 to 8 years	1.5 mg
Males 9 to 13 years	1.9 mg
Males 14 to 18 years	2.2 mg
Males 19 years and older	2.3 mg
Females 9 to 18 years	1.6 mg
Females 19 years and older	1.8 mg
Pregnant females	2 mg
Lactating females	2.6 mg

* Regulation of blood sugar levels
* Protein synthesis
* Healthy cardiovascular system
* Nerve functions
* Strong bones
* Synthesis of DNA and RNA
* Transport of calcium and potassium
* Muscle contraction

DEFICIENCY AND TOXICITY

Since magnesium plays such a crucial role, a magnesium deficiency is very damaging and affects every system in the body. Besides dietary deficiencies, certain conditions such as chronic alcoholism, Crohn's disease, and type 2 diabetes can also lead to magnesium losses that exceed healthy levels. Symptoms of a magnesium deficiency can include:

* Abnormal heart rhythms
* Anxiety
* Calcium deficiency
* Difficulty swallowing
* Dizziness
* Fatigue
* High blood pressure
* Loss of appetite
* Muscle contractions
* Muscle cramps
* Nausea
* Numbness
* Personality changes
* Poor memory
* Potassium deficiency
* Respiratory issues
* Seizures
* Tremors
* Vomiting

Chronic low levels of magnesium are thought to lead to an increased risk of cardiovascular disease, osteoporosis, and diabetes. A series of studies in several different countries with thousands of subjects indicates that higher magnesium levels decrease the risk of stroke, ischemic heart disease, and sudden cardiac death. Other studies seem to point to an increase in bone mineral density when people take magnesium supplements. The American Diabetes Association does not endorse magnesium as a proven method to control blood sugar, but statistics from population studies indicate that there might be a benefit. For example, data compiled from seven studies spanning six to seventeen years and involving 286,668 patients found that the risk of diabetes decreased 15 percent with magnesium supplements of 100 mg per day. This data on magnesium is significant enough to warrant further testing.

Magnesium toxicity is not common in healthy people. Magnesium can build up to unsafe levels in people with kidney disease because this condition interferes with normal elimination of this mineral. Long-term antacid or laxative users, and those who take supplementary magnesium, can also experience magnesium toxicity. The symptoms of excess magnesium often manifest first as diarrhea, nausea, cramps, and vomiting. Other symptoms include low blood pressure, irregular heartbeat, depression, breathing issues, muscle weakness, confusion, fatigue, and, with extreme toxicity, cardiac arrest, coma, or death.

RECOMMENDED AMOUNTS AND FOODS

Magnesium is plentiful in the food chain, and foods with lots of fiber usually contain magnesium. Sources of magnesium include dark leafy greens, legumes, whole grains, nuts and seeds, squash, quinoa, bananas, avocados, tuna, scallops, papaya, beets, broccoli, tofu, almonds, Brussels sprouts, raspberries, tomatoes, cabbage, strawberries, and bok choy. Magnesium is also available as a supplement, which you might see labeled as magnesium citrate, chloride, and oxide. Magnesium is the main ingredient in heartburn medication and laxatives such as milk of magnesia or Rolaids.

Most people in the United States (about 75 percent of the population) do not get enough magnesium in their diets. People who use magnesium supplements and medications usually have adequate levels. According to

minerals

RDA: MAGNESIUM

The RDA for magnesium is as follows:

0 to 6 months	30 mg
7 to 12 months	75 mg
1 to 3 years	80 mg
9 to 13 years	240 mg
14 to 18 years	360 mg
Males 19 years and older	400 mg
Females 19 to 30 years	310 mg
Females 31 years and older	320 mg
Pregnant females up to 30 years	350 mg
Lactating females up to 30 years	310 mg
Pregnant females 31 and older	360 mg
Lactating females 31 and older	320 mg

the National Health and Nutrition Examination Survey, the average total intakes with supplements are 449 mg per day for men and 387 mg per day for women.

MOLYBDENUM

Molybdenum is a trace element that is necessary for the human body to function. When ingested, molybdenum is quickly absorbed in the stomach and small intestine. It travels through the blood in red blood cells and, bound to alpha-macro globulin, to the liver and other tissues. In the liver, a molybdenum atom is bound to tricyclic pyranapterin molecules and a molybdenum cofactor is formed, which is a crucial component of four enzymes:

* Aldehyde oxidase, which is involved in many reactions, including the breakdown of pyrimidines
* Sulfite oxidase, which brings about the conversion of sulfite to sulfate; crucial for the metabolism of amino acids that contain sulfur
* Xanthine dehydrogenase, which is responsible for the conversion of xanthine to uric acid and hypoxanthine to xanthine
* Xanthine oxidase, which increases the antioxidant capacity of the blood by bringing about the breakdown of nucleotides to form uric acid

These enzymes also help metabolize fats, carbohydrates, toxins, and drugs as well as remove iron from the liver and prevent tooth decay. High levels of molybdenum can create a copper deficiency, because molybdenum can block copper absorption. Therapies using a compound called ammonium tetrathiomolybdate can treat conditions relating to copper accumulation in the body, such as Wilson's disease. Since copper-dependent enzymes can accelerate cancer metastasis, studies are also looking at molybdenum therapies to prevent the advancement of malignancies.

DEFICIENCY AND TOXICITY
Molybdenum deficiency is rare in healthy people living in areas that have this element in the soil. Areas deficient in molybdenum, such as China,

see a higher incidence of esophageal cancer, but the link is not conclusive. Molybdenum deficiency is seen in patients on long-term feeding IVs without molybdenum supplementation, and manifests as high levels of urate and sulfite in the blood. These damaging levels cause night blindness, headaches, rapid heart rate, and coma. This decline in patient health can be reversed when molybdenum is administered. Other forms of molybdenum deficiency occur in an inherited disease called molybdenum cofactor deficiency, which causes mental retardation, seizures, and cerebral atrophy. This disease usually results in death in early childhood because molybdenum-dependent enzymes are not available. Molybdenum cofactor deficiency is extremely rare, with only about 100 people affected worldwide.

Molybdenum toxicity is not common. There is limited research on excessive molybdenum amounts in humans, but studies on rats show that very high doses can cause low birth weight, diarrhea, infertility, gout, and stunted growth. One human case showed that supplementing 13.5 mg per day of molybdenum over 18 days caused hallucinations, neurological symptoms, and seizures. The symptoms disappeared over the course of several hours when the patient was treated with chelation therapy. Workers exposed to high levels of molybdenum in copper-molybdenum plants show an increase in gout and uric acid levels in the blood, as well as loss of appetite, fatigue, muscle pain, and headaches.

RECOMMENDED AMOUNTS AND FOOD SOURCES

The amount of molybdenum in your food depends on the soil where it is grown. Since molybdenum is plentiful in North American soil, getting enough molybdenum in your diet is not difficult. Some of the best sources of molybdenum are legumes, whole grains, nuts, eggs, pork, beef liver, lamb, green beans, sunflower seeds, cucumbers, dark green leafy vegetables, milk, tomatoes, carrots, yogurt, and cottage cheese. A Food and Drug Administration (FDA) report that outlines the mineral content in the typical US diet shows that the daily intake of molybdenum typically is above the recommended amount, with men getting 109 mcg and women getting 76 mcg.

minerals

RDA: MOLYBDENUM

The daily RDA for molybdenum is as follows:

0 to 6 months	2 mcg
7 to 11 months	3 mcg
1 to 3 years	17 mcg
4 to 8 years	22 mcg
9 to 13 years	34 mcg
14 to 18 years	43 mcg
19 years and older	45 mcg
Pregnant and lactating females	50 mcg

SELENIUM

Selenium is an essential element. It is a component of about 24 selenoproteins that are crucial for protection from free radicals, reproduction, and the metabolism of thyroid hormones. These selenoproteins can be found in the blood, organs, testicles, prostate gland, and cell membranes. Selenium is absorbed easily in the gut. The amounts not required for bodily functions are excreted within about 24 hours through the urine, feces, and breath.

One of the most important purposes of selenoproteins is to prevent oxidative stress from free radicals. The group of selenoproteins responsible for this antioxidant activity is called the glutathione peroxidases. These selenoproteins also boost antioxidant protection by recycling vitamin C from an inactive into an active form. Glutathione peroxidase has another crucial function: it inactivates the hydrogen peroxide generated in the thyroid gland. Hydrogen peroxide occurs when a protein called thyroglobulin connects tyrosine and iodine to create the thyroid hormone T_4. If the hydrogen peroxide is not inactivated, the thyroid is damaged and thyroid hormones are not produced in sufficient amounts. T_4 is activated and deactivated by other selenoproteins, so selenium is crucial for regulating this hormone.

Selenoproteins also:

* Play a role in producing white blood cells
* Support a healthy reproductive system
* Promote healthy liver function
* Help metabolize fats
* Support glowing skin and strong hair
* Promote a healthy cardiovascular system

DEFICIENCY AND TOXICITY

Selenium deficiency is rare in North America, but some people in some other countries do have selenium deficiencies, especially if the predominant diet is vegetable-based and the soil is low in selenium. A selenium deficiency contributes to the development of conditions and diseases such as Kashin-Beck disease and Keshan disease, which are linked with selenium deficiency combined with viral infections or infertility. The risk of cretinism in infants is increased when iodine deficiency is exacerbated by a selenium deficiency. When patients with HIV have low levels of selenium, their risk of death and cardiomyopathy is higher. Selenium deficiency is also linked inconclusively to an increased risk of cancer, but more research is needed at this point.

Excessive selenium is more of an issue in areas with abundant selenium in the water and soil. People may also overdose when they supplement too much. If the exposure to selenium occurs over the long term or is particularly high, excess selenium can build up in the liver, kidneys, lungs, heart, blood, nails, and hair. The symptoms of excessive selenium include:

* Brittle hair or hair loss
* A metallic taste in the mouth
* Weak nails
* Garlic breath (without eating garlic)
* Skin rashes
* Tooth discoloration or decay
* Fatigue
* Headaches
* Vomiting and nausea
* Diarrhea
* Irritability
* Nervous system abnormalities
* Kidney failure
* Cardiac arrest
* Death (in severe cases)

When excessive amounts of selenium are inhaled, the effects are centered on the respiratory system and include coughing, nosebleeds, irritated mucous membranes, bronchitis, difficulty breathing, and pneumonia.

RECOMMENDED AMOUNTS AND FOOD SOURCES

The amount of selenium in food is influenced by environmental factors. In North America, commercially raised animals are given selenium supplements; eggs, chicken, beef, and pork all contain high levels of the mineral.

minerals

RDA: SELENIUM

The daily RDA for selenium per day is as follows:

0 to 6 months	15 mcg
7 to 12 months	20 mcg
1 to 3 years	20 mcg
4 to 8 years	30 mcg
9 to 13 years	40 mcg
14 to 18 years	55 mcg
19 years and older	55 mcg
Pregnant females	60 mcg
Lactating females	70 mcg

Fruits and vegetables contain different levels of selenium depending on their growing zones. Dietary sources of selenium include Brazil nuts, organ meats, seafood, whole grains, poultry, eggs, meat, dairy, green peas, carrots, asparagus, flaxseed, lettuce, bananas, tofu, potatoes, mushrooms, sesame seeds, spinach, lentils, garlic, and cashews.

Most people get adequate amounts of selenium through dietary sources. Selenium is also an ingredient in most multivitamins. The average selenium intake in the United States is estimated to be about 110 mcg from food sources alone, and about 120 mcg if supplemented. These intakes differ depending on location, because soil concentrations of selenium vary.

SILICON

Silicon is the second most common element on earth. Silicon represents about 1 percent of human body weight and is found in the skin, blood vessels, cartilage, tendons, and bones. Silicon provides stability and strength, so it is essential for helping to strengthen connective tissues in the human body.

This element has been the subject of recent research that studies its impact on human health. It is known that silicon takes part in the formation of connective tissue in the body, and that the amount of silicon in areas of the body such as the aorta, thymus, and skin decreases as people age. This might contribute to the formation of arteriosclerosis and wrinkles. The amount of silicon in the skin, hair, and tooth enamel is substantial, which has led to hypotheses about silicon playing a role in protecting these areas by being a barrier. A study testing the effects of applying silicon as a topical treatment has yielded results that suggest silicon improves the thickness and strength of skin, and increases the health of nails and hair. Silicon has also been linked to preventing the onset of osteoporosis and osteoarthritis by contributing to the repair and formation of bones. Silicon can keep bones healthy and slow the progression of bone-related illnesses. Silicon is often a recommended supplement for people with bone illness.

DEFICIENCY AND TOXICITY
Silicon deficiency is quite rare because of the availability of this mineral in dietary choices. The only reason some people take silicon supplements

is to treat osteoporosis. Silicon deficiency affects areas of the body that require healthy connective tissue, so low levels cause brittle nails, brittle hair, premature aging, wrinkles, and weakened bones and cartilage. Silicon deficiency can also contribute to damaged blood vessels, a condition that facilitates cholesterol buildup and increases the risk of atherosclerosis. Some research indicates that silicon can boost physical endurance and, since silicon can block the absorption of aluminum in the brain to some extent, it is thought that low levels of silicon can decrease the risk of Alzheimer's disease. Excessive silicon exposure is rare but can cause digestive issues, skin problems, and bruising.

RECOMMENDED AMOUNTS AND FOOD SOURCES

Most people should be able to meet their silicon needs through diet, as this mineral is found in many foods. Silicon is an important component in plant fibers and helps prevent stalks from wilting, toughens leaves, and can even ward off damaging pests. Excellent sources of this mineral are whole grains with hulls, bananas, leafy greens, sugar beets, alfalfa, onions, lettuce, parsnips, celery, apples, dandelions, strawberries, grapes, peanuts, raw almonds, oranges, raisins, carrots, raw sunflower seeds, beans, lentils, avocados, string beans, pumpkin, fish, raw flaxseed, organ meats, mussels, and beer. There is also silicon in hard water and coffee. Silicon is easily lost in processing, such as in making flour from wheat, so the best sources of this element are whole foods.

There is no RDA for silicon, and advice from various health agencies varies, recommending dosages from 5 to 50 mg daily. The absorption rate of silicon is not understood, and the upper number is meant to ensure adequate silicon is available in the body. Silicon is mainly absorbed in the gastrointestinal tract, and the amount taken in depends on the form consumed. Plant-derived silicon is thought to be generally unavailable, because it is in an insoluble form such as fiber. The most biologically available form of silicon can be found in beer and hard water. A high calcium and magnesium diet can have a detrimental effect on silicon uptake. Most people get about 20 to 50 mg per day through dietary sources.

SODIUM

Sodium is an essential mineral that is crucial for life. Salt is formed when sodium combines with chloride. Sodium is an electrolyte, a positively charged cation, formed when salts dissolve in a fluid. There is more sodium outside the cells than inside, where potassium is the principal cation. Studies have shown that between 20 and 40 percent of resting energy of the body goes toward regulating sodium and potassium concentrations across the cell membranes (called membrane potential). Membrane potential must be perfectly balanced for nerve transmission, cardiac health, and muscle contraction. Sodium and chloride are responsible for the volume of fluid outside the cells, including blood plasma. This means that sodium plays a role in blood pressure, regulation of the pH of the blood, and waste removal from cells. Balance is necessary for normal blood volume: high sodium is mirrored by water retention, and low sodium results in water loss. If the blood volume increases due to water retention, the blood vessels cannot expand to accommodate the excess, and high blood pressure will occur. If sodium is not adequately regulated by the kidneys, brain, and endocrine glands, death can result.

DEFICIENCY AND TOXICITY

Sodium deficiency is often not a serious concern. Even very-low-salt diets do not usually produce any health issues. When, however, serum sodium concentration reaches less than 136 mmol/liter, a condition called hyponatremia arises. You can lose sodium with excessive sweating, severe vomiting or diarrhea, kidney disease, and during prolonged endurance exercise. Hyponatremia symptoms include fainting, confusion, vomiting, nausea, headache, muscle cramps, and fatigue. Certain medications such as diuretics, antidepressants, NSAIDs, and opiates can also cause hyponatremia. If left untreated, severe hyponatremia can lead to swelling of the brain, brain damage, seizures, coma, and death.

Excess sodium is an issue today thanks to our reliance on processed foods. Hypertension, or high blood pressure, can occur when the intake of dietary sodium is too high. High blood pressure increases the risk of heart attack, stroke, and kidney disease because it damages the blood vessels, heart, and kidneys. Other diseases linked to chronic high-sodium diets include osteoporosis, stomach cancer, and kidney stones. When the sodium levels in the blood are too high, exceeding 145 mmol/liter, a condition called hypernatremia occurs. Hypernatremia is usually not due to diet, but rather can be caused by extreme water restriction, severe diarrhea, hormone imbalance, untreated diabetes, and kidney disease. The symptoms of hypernatremia are irregular heartbeat, fainting, extreme thirst, sunken eyes, fatigue, dark urine, muscle spasms, seizures, and coma.

RECOMMENDED AMOUNTS AND FOOD SOURCES

Sodium occurs naturally in most foods. Some foods, such as shrimp, spinach, Swiss chard, artichokes, cantaloupe, celery, and seaweed contain high amounts of the mineral. Salt is the most common source of sodium and chloride in most people's diets. Table salt is about 40 percent sodium by weight. The sodium added during processing and cooking usually makes up about 75 percent of the sodium in a product, so reading nutrition labels is crucial. Foods that are high in sodium include:

* Canned and frozen foods
* Processed meats
* Breads
* Cheeses
* Pickled foods
* Pasta sauces
* Condiments
* Cereals
* Snack foods
* Tomato juice

Some research indicates that human beings can remain healthy and have their sodium needs met by absorbing 500 mg per day, or less than 1/4 teaspoon. However, the adequate intake levels set by the National Academy of Sciences are higher and take into account the amount of sodium lost in sweat during moderate exercise and in urine.

RDA: SODIUM

The recommended adequate intake per day for sodium is as follows:

0 to 6 months	120 mg
7 to 12 months	370 mg
1 to 3 years	1,000 mg
4 to 8 years	1,200 mg
9 to 50 years	1,500 mg
50 to 70 years	1,300 mg
71 years and older	1,200 mg
Pregnant and lactating females	1,500 mg

"SNAKE OILS"

Almost every day there seems to emerge some new super supplement that's supposed to miraculously strip years from your skin and make you lose all the pounds you want without even trying. If it seems too good to be true, it probably is. Most of these miracle claims don't come from science; they come from marketers, and they are very likely either completely untrue or gross exaggerations. Some manufacturers of these snake oils will commission "studies" that include the right scientific lingo but massage the data to present the product in a beneficial light. Be wary of grandiose promises. There's no miracle food or supplement that will instantly make you healthier. Instead, that requires a long-term commitment to healthy eating.

SULFUR

Sulfur is considered to be an essential mineral and is stored in every cell in the body, especially the muscles, hair, joints, and skin. Adults store approximately 140 g of sulfur in the body, mostly in the form of amino acids such as cysteine and methionine. Dietary sources of sulfur are needed to replenish its supply in the body, because sulfur is used daily by the body for an array of functions. Excess amounts of sulfur are either stored as glutathione, an antioxidant, or excreted through urine. Sulfur plays many roles in the body because it is a component of amino acids, protein, insulin, heparin, taurine, biotin, coenzyme A, glutathione, lipoic acid, thiamine, hemoglobin, enzymes, antibodies, and glycosaminoglycans. Some of the functions and processes in the body that sulfur is essential for include:

* Forming collagen
* Maintaining and strengthening skin, hair, and nails as a component of keratin
* Regulating carbohydrate metabolism
* Helping to regulate blood sugar
* Helping cells utilize oxygen
* Aiding brain function
* Aiding the liver to eliminate toxins and produce bile
* Aiding in digestion
* Promoting healthy joints
* Strengthening cell walls
* Helping to regulate nerves
* Lowering inflammation
* Slowing nerve impulses that transmit pain signals
* Serving as a component of bones, cartilage, and tendons
* Building healthy elastic blood vessels
* Burning fat
* Protecting cells from free radicals

DEFICIENCY AND TOXICITY

Sulfur deficiency is rare, because most people get enough in their diet unless they are strict vegans, live in an area with mineral-depleted soil, or have an underlying medical condition that interferes with sulfur absorption. Sulfur deficiencies are usually associated with low concentrations of methylsulfonylmethane (MSM) in the body, which is an organic source of sulfur found in plants. The symptoms of MSM deficiency are:

* Acne
* Arthritis
* Brittle hair
* Brittle nails
* Circulation issues
* Constipation
* Convulsions
* Degenerative diseases
* Depression
* Fatigue
* Gastrointestinal challenges
* Inflammation
* Memory loss
* Muscle pain
* Nerve disorders
* Rashes
* Scar tissue
* Slow wound healing
* Stress
* Wrinkles

Sulfur toxicity is not a common issue for people with no sensitivities to this mineral. Excessive ingestion of sulfur supplements can cause digestive issues. Long-term exposure to high levels of sulfur is linked to calcium and potassium deficiencies, impaired immune response, and more acute allergy symptoms. People with Crohn's disease or Lou Gehrig's disease can find that their symptoms worsen if they take too much sulfur. This mineral can also be taken in via inorganic sources such as food additives, medications, fossil fuel emissions, and pesticides.

RECOMMENDED AMOUNTS AND FOOD SOURCES

The best sources of sulfur are animal-based proteins, such as meat, poultry, eggs (especially the yolks), fish, milk, and cheese. Vegans can sometimes suffer from a sulfur deficiency because they do not consume the richest sources of this mineral. However, there are vegan choices that are good sources of sulfur, including onions, garlic, Brussels sprouts, kale, kelp, raspberries, turnips, cabbage, legumes, jicama, nuts, sesame seeds, sunflower seeds, coconut, broccoli, bananas, mustard greens, pineapple, asparagus, sweet potatoes, avocados, cauliflower, tomatoes, coffee, tea, cocoa, and watermelon. People can also get sulfur from sulfites, a common food preservative. Sulfites, however, may trigger an immune response in the body and are not considered to be a nutrient.

Even though sulfur is one of the most plentiful minerals in the body, there is no official RDA. This is puzzling, as sulfur is almost completely obtained from dietary sources, especially protein. You can usually get an adequate amount if you are also meeting your protein needs, but a healthy sulfur level for an adult is about 1 g per day, and 5 g as a short-term therapeutic dose.

TIN

Tin is a trace mineral that can be found in small amounts in the body, especially in the suprarenal glands, brain, liver, thyroid gland, and spleen. Researchers are not sure exactly how necessary tin is to good health because it is not found in newborns or many animals, but some studies indicate that this mineral merits a closer look. Many rat studies show that these animals do not grow well on a low-tin diet, and suffer hearing loss, hair loss, and a diminished appetite. Rats fed a diet higher in tin fell into normal physical and anatomical ranges. Studies concerning the impact of tin on human beings are not prevalent, although a two-year study on 285 humans demonstrated that tin can provide some health benefits. One result of the study was that tin did not have any negative impact, and that participants reported feeling better physically. Some of the positive health reports to come out of the study include improvements in skin issues, fatigue, mood, depression, digestion, and pain. There was also a marked decrease in the frequency of insomnia, asthma, and headaches for many participants.

Iodine supports the thyroid and tin supports the adrenals. Researchers have noted that a combined deficiency in vitamin C, vitamin B, and tin can cause low adrenals, which can lead to left-side heart issues. This issue, in turn, results in asthma and breathing problems.

DEFICIENCY AND TOXICITY

Most people will get 1 to 3 mg of tin per day from food and water if they do not eat canned foods. Lacquered tin-lined cans containing 600 g of acidic contents can increase tin intake by 15 mg per can, and before cans were lined, a can of tomatoes could increase intake by 60 mg. It is difficult to tell how much of the 1 to 3 mg of tin actually crosses into the blood from the intestinal tract, because tin is so poorly absorbed—probably at a rate of only 5 percent. Any excess tin is eliminated through the feces, urine, and perspiration. Since not much is known about the impact of tin on the body, it is probably prudent to avoid excessive or long-term exposure. There have been cases of tin toxicity when food and drinks were stored in cans made from tin and people were exposed to hundreds of milligrams of this mineral. The symptoms of tin toxicity are mostly gastrointestinal in nature, such as vomiting, nausea, diarrhea, and cramps, but since this mineral is excreted so quickly, no long-term health issues were reported. Tin deficiency is a less studied condition, although there are studies outlining the effects of tin deficiency in animals. Tin deficiency in people can manifest as depression, low adrenals, insomnia, headache, and shortness of breath.

RECOMMENDED AMOUNTS AND FOOD SOURCES

Tin is absorbed from the growing environment, so almost all fruits and vegetables contain a trace amount. The quantity of the mineral in food depends on how much tin there is in the soil. Other sources of tin can be found in canned foods, meat, dairy, seaweed, cereal grains, and brewer's yeast.

There is currently no RDA for tin put forth as essential to health, but a guideline to consider is 1 to 5 mg daily for children up to age 10, and 10 to 20 mg daily for those 11 years and older.

VANADIUM

Vanadium is considered to be an essential trace element, but more research needs to be conducted on its effects. Vanadium is found in the soil, and the amount present influences how much of this element ends up in the food that grows in the soil. When ingested, 5 to 10 percent of vanadium is absorbed. Vanadium is used rapidly in the body and then excreted in the urine if not needed. Any unabsorbed vanadium is eliminated in the feces. Vanadium is stored in tiny amounts all over the body, about 20 to 25 mg in total, especially in the fat tissue.

Vanadium acts similarly to insulin in the body, which indicates that it could be a solution for people with conditions related to glucose, such as diabetes. Vanadium makes the cell membrane more receptive to glucose so that glucose is transported and stored more readily, in addition to activating glycogen synthesis and facilitating the storage of glycogen in the muscles. Research into the effects of vanadium on diabetes is geared toward finding treatments less invasive than injections of insulin. In studies, rats showed near-normal blood sugar levels with no weight gain when administered a vanadium-based insulin mimic known as bis (maltolato) oxovanadium (IV).

Early work with vanadium in the 1960s linked this element to both lipid metabolism and a decrease in cholesterol levels. This suggests that vanadium might be an effective treatment for high cholesterol and related conditions, such as atherosclerosis and cardiovascular disease. The anticarcinogenic properties of vanadium are of interest to many researchers, as studies have found that vanadium can reduce the incidence, size, and number of tumors in mice, particularly in mammary tissue. This element does not negatively affect the animal's health, making it a possible substitution for chemotherapy and radiation in the future. Other animal studies involve looking at vanadium with respect to growth, calcium metabolism, red blood cell production, bone formation, and reproduction, but no conclusive results have been reported yet.

DEFICIENCY AND TOXICITY

Most of the data on vanadium deficiency needs to be substantiated with more research before definitive conclusions can be drawn. Animal studies have yielded some possible issues such as birth defects in the bones and premature death in babies from mothers fed a vanadium-deficient diet, an increased risk of heart disease and cancer, and a decrease in growth. Conditions that have been linked to a vanadium deficiency in animal studies include diabetes, infertility, hypoglycemia, cardiovascular disease, obesity, and hyperglycemia.

Since vanadium is not absorbed well, this essential trace element is thought to be generally nontoxic, although excess quantities in the body could be dangerous, as evidenced in animal studies. Some of the issues associated with toxic levels of vanadium in animals are diarrhea, high blood pressure, a decrease in coenzyme Q_{10} and coenzyme A levels, impaired energy production in cells, and changes in monoamine oxidase inhibitors. The only human indicator of potential issues related to excessive vanadium is the fact that high levels of this element are present in people who have bipolar disorder.

RECOMMENDED AMOUNTS AND FOOD SOURCES

The vanadium needs of the body are thought to be met by diet, but this is difficult to determine because there is no RDA for this element. Most diets provide about 2 mg per day, which is more than adequate to meet nutritional demands. Diets high in fish and fish oils can bump that amount up to 10 or 15 mg per day. Dietary sources of vanadium include black pepper, dill seeds, whole grains, parsley, sunflower oil, mushrooms, buckwheat, peanut butter, shellfish, herring, seafood, oats, rice, olive oil, dairy products, chicken breast, green beans, radish, carrots, eggs, and cabbage.

minerals

ZINC

Zinc is an important trace mineral necessary for good health. It also works as a cofactor with a number of enzymes. Zinc naturally occurs in foods and is found in cells throughout the body.

This mineral helps your immune system work properly. In fact, zinc lozenges can be effective in fighting colds. Studies show that when taken within 24 hours of developing symptoms, zinc lozenges can help reduce the severity and duration of the cold virus. People with a zinc deficiency may experience weakened immunity as zinc improves the ability of your T-cells to function.

Zinc plays a key role in cell growth and proliferation. Research shows that children need adequate zinc in their diets to achieve expected standards of height and weight. The mineral is especially important for normal development of reproductive organs and the brain.

A diet containing adequate amounts of zinc is essential for healthy brain function as the mineral aids signaling between neurons. In children, diets low in zinc may also contribute to behavioral and learning issues.

DEFICIENCY AND TOXICITY

Because zinc is essential in cell function throughout the body, deficiency may cause a number of issues. Problems arising from zinc deficiency include:

* Loss of sense of smell and taste
* Loss of appetite
* Brain fog
* Poor cognitive function
* Decreased immunity
* Persistent and frequent infections
* Delayed growth and development in children
* Patchy hair loss
* Decreased sperm production in men
* Night blindness
* Poor or incomplete wound healing
* Rashes
* Birth defects or low birth weight, if the mother is deficient in zinc

While zinc deficiency can be associated with inadequate zinc intake from dietary sources, it can also occur as a result of malabsorption syndromes, such as untreated celiac disease. Zinc deficiency can also have genetic causes or be related to factors such as excessive alcohol intake, the use of certain drugs and medications, and kidney and liver diseases.

Zinc toxicity is possible, but usually arises from supplementation and not from consuming foods high in zinc. Symptoms may include loss of appetite, vomiting, nausea, and stomach pain. Supplementing too much zinc may also block absorption of other important minerals, such as copper and iron.

Sometimes taking zinc supplements is necessary, but be sure to work with your health care provider. Not only can zinc be toxic, it can also interact with certain medications. For example, zinc significantly reduces the absorption of penicillamine. Likewise, zinc can interact with quinolone and tetracycline antibiotics, reducing absorption of both the medication and the zinc.

RECOMMENDED AMOUNTS AND FOOD SOURCES

Because zinc occurs mostly in animal sources, vegetarians and vegans may be at risk of deficiency and should ensure they eat foods containing adequate zinc or talk with their health care provider about taking a zinc supplement. A number of foods are excellent sources of zinc. These foods include:

* Mollusks, such as oysters and clams
* Beef
* Crustaceans, such as crab and lobster
* Chicken
* Lamb
* Fish
* Cashews
* Garbanzo beans
* Oats
* Cheese
* Peas

minerals

RDA: ZINC

The RDA for zinc varies for each age group:

0 to 6 months	2mg
7 months to 3 years	3mg
4 to 8 years require	5 mg
9 to13 years	8mg
Males 14 years and older	11mg
Females 14 to 18 years	9mg
Females 19 years and older	8mg
Pregnant women	11 to 12mg
Lactating women	12 to 13 mg

Over half of the volume of your body is made up of water. It is integrated into every piece of you, and it plays a vital role in every single part and process of your body. Next to air, water is the most important substance you provide your body with. In fact, you can live for only about eight days without water.

water

WHERE THE WATER GOES

Different parts of your body are thirstier than others. For example, your skin is about 64 percent water, while your brain and heart are composed of about 73 percent water. Even your bones contain more than 30 percent of their volume in water.

WHAT THE WATER DOES

Water plays so many roles in your body that it is essential to life itself. In the body, water:

* is a building block for cells, assisting in cell reproduction and growth, and forming part of the cell's structure.
* regulates your body temperature, helping to keep you within a safe and healthy range. For example, when you get too hot, you sweat.
* plays a vital role in digestion, helping to convert food to energy and nutrients. It is also part of saliva, which starts the process of breakdown as you chew and swallow your foods.
* is used to manufacture chemicals in the brain, such as neurotransmitters and hormones.
* transports micro- and macronutrients in the bloodstream to every cell in your body.
* protects your organs, nerves, and bones, and provides a cushion for your spinal cord.
* carries oxygen to every cell in your body.
* helps flush waste products that your body does not need, via sweat and urine.
* protects the developing fetus as a part of amniotic fluid.
* keeps your joints from getting creaky by forming synovial fluid, which provides lubrication and cushioning.
* keeps all of your mucous membranes, such as your eyes, moist and supple.

HOW MUCH YOU NEED

A number of factors determine how much water you need on a daily basis. Factors affecting your water needs include:

* Age
* Sex
* Body weight
* Activity level
* Ambient temperature
* Sweating

In general, a male adult needs approximately 3 liters of water each day, while an adult female needs around 2.2 liters. If you are highly active, if you sweat a lot, or if you are in a very hot climate, you may require more water. Likewise, if you have diarrhea or are vomiting, you may need to drink more to replenish your fluids.

You do not need to carefully measure your water to make sure you have enough, however. If your urine is light in color, not dark, then you're probably adequately hydrated.

WATER AND ELECTROLYTES

In your body, water mixes with other chemicals and fluids, including electrolytes. The water and electrolytes in your body coexist in a delicate balance, and the body does everything it can to maintain this balance.

Electrolytes are minerals that have an electrical charge. They cause the contraction and relaxation of every muscle in your body, including your heart. When you have too much water in your system, your electrolytes may become diluted and inefficient. When you have too little water, your electrolytes may become too concentrated.

To a great extent, your body maintains this delicate balance very well, holding onto water when the concentration gets a little high, and excreting water when the electrolytes are too dilute. Sometimes extreme conditions may affect this delicate balance. These may include intense exercise, extremely hot weather, drinking a lot very quickly, vomiting, and diarrhea.

water

ELECTROLYTES

Electrolytes are minerals in the body that have an electrical charge. They control muscle relaxation and contraction, including your heartbeat. Electrolyte imbalances can have mild effects, such as muscle cramping, or severe effects, such as heart arrhythmia. In extreme circumstances, such as when you engage in intense physical exercise, when you are vomiting or having diarrhea, or when you sweat a great deal, you may lose electrolytes rapidly. In these cases, you may wish to replace them with an electrolyte solution. However, in normal circumstances, your body maintains a relatively steady balance of electrolytes. Eating a balanced diet can ensure your body has the electrolytes it needs for healthy function.

DEHYDRATION

Dehydration can have a number of effects on the body. It can cause a loss of energy and lethargy. It can also make you feel hungry when in fact you're thirsty. You may also notice brain fog, muscle cramping, and changes in mood. Fortunately, the effects of mild dehydration can easily be reversed by drinking water. Severe dehydration, however, may require medical intervention. To prevent dehydration, drink when you're thirsty and try to sip water throughout the day.

HYPONATREMIA

In some cases, when you drink very large amounts of water too quickly for your body to excrete, you risk a rare condition called hyponatremia, when the water in your body dilutes your electrolytes so much that your cells start swelling. Symptoms may include nausea, confusion, energy loss, or muscle weakness. The condition can be mild, or it may be life-threatening.

SOURCES OF WATER

You do not have to drink 3 liters of water each day to meet your body's requirement. You get water in just about everything you consume, including other beverages. There's even water in your food that will contribute to your body's overall water content.

Of course, the best source of water is pure water. Drinking six or seven cups per day will keep you adequately hydrated.

TAP WATER

In most places, tap water is perfectly safe. The water from your tap is not pure water. Instead, it also contains trace minerals and elements that are perfectly safe. The mineral content of your water depends on where you live. Some municipal suppliers may add fluoride to the local water supply. However, the Environmental Protection Agency has regulations in place to protect the safety of your tap water, requiring your municipal water supplier to provide a report every year about the source and contents of your water.

WELL WATER

Well water is not regulated by any agency. Therefore, it is important that if you drink water from a well on your property, you have it tested for quality and safety every year.

BOTTLED WATER

The FDA regulates bottled water, ensuring sanitation and safety. While some bottled waters come from wells or springs, others come from the tap where they are bottled. Therefore, there is no guarantee that bottled water is any safer than tap or well water.

There is also some concern about the bottles in which the water comes. According to the Natural Resources Defense Council, plastic water bottles may contain phthalates, which are hormone disrupters. These chemicals may leach into the water that comes in the bottles.

Large, hard plastic (polycarbonate) water bottles in dispensers may contain bisphenol A, or BPA, which may mimic the hormone estrogen. This may disrupt hormones or lead to other problems. Research into the safety of BPA is ongoing.

SODA, JUICE, ALCOHOL, AND OTHER SOURCES OF WATER
Many people primarily drink their liquids in the form of coffee, tea, soda, juice, and energy drinks. While these beverages do contain water and can help serve your body's hydration needs, they may have other issues associated with them.

For example, drinks that contain caffeine, such as coffee, tea, energy drinks, and sodas, may have a diuretic effect on the body. This causes your body to lose water, which may dehydrate you and make your water requirements increase.

Likewise, sugar serves as a diuretic and has other negative effects on the body (see page 49), including causing elevated levels of glucose. Many of these drinks also serve as a source of empty calories, providing your body with energy without nutrition. This can cause weight gain.

Alcohol can also dehydrate you by causing diuresis (excessive urination).

Finally, even if you are drinking decaffeinated, artificially sweetened sodas or energy drinks, you are providing your body with a host of foreign chemicals it may not be able to process. Artificial sweeteners, while non-caloric, may actually increase hunger and cravings for sugar. Studies have linked consumption of artificial sweeteners like sucralose and aspartame to weight gain.

The bottom line is this: drink clear, clean water and minimize your intake of other sources of fluid, such as coffee, tea, soda, alcohol, and energy drinks.

water

antioxidants

The metabolism of oxygen in the body creates free radicals, which are compounds that remove electrons from healthy molecules, causing damage and deterioration. This condition is called oxidative stress. Antioxidants are substances that fight or decrease the effects of oxidative stress in the body.

FREE RADICALS

These free radicals may provide pathways for degeneration and disease, and they are also the primary cause of aging. Free radicals can damage cells and DNA.

A number of factors can increase the amount of free radicals your body produces and the oxidative stress it encounters. These include:

* Smoking
* Heavy alcohol consumption
* Cooking fats and oils at very high temperatures or consuming oxidized fats and oils
* Consuming highly processed foods
* Consuming processed meats
* Cooking meats at very high temperatures

ANTIOXIDANTS TO THE RESCUE

Free radicals can do a lot of damage in the body, but there is something that can counteract their effects: antioxidants. These substances can delay or counteract the damage caused by free radicals. Substances that work as antioxidants in your body include vitamins A, C, and E, beta-carotene, lutein, and lycopene.

AGING

Since free radicals and oxidative stress play such a large role in aging, antioxidants may help slow this process. A correlation exists between consumption of a high level of antioxidants and longevity in mammals. Studies have shown that consumption of a diet high in antioxidants helps delay or prevent the onset of age-related diseases, such as macular degeneration and dementia.

CANCER

Studies show that antioxidants fight free radical damage that may lead to certain types of cancer, according to the National Cancer Institute. However, in general, the results of these studies have been mixed. As previously mentioned, supplementation of some antioxidants, such as vitamin E, has actually been associated to an increased risk of cancer. Therefore, supplementation may not be the answer, whereas eating foods high in antioxidants can help as part of an overall disease prevention plan.

HEART DISEASE

Research at the Cleveland Clinic has examined the role of antioxidants in heart disease. It is believed that free radical damage is at least partially responsible for LDL cholesterol becoming atherosclerotic and sticking to the lining of blood vessels. Research has shown that, while vitamin E supplementation doesn't seem to affect heart disease, beta-carotene supplementation actually increased the risk of all-cause mortality slightly. However, this applies to supplements only. Eating healthy foods that contain antioxidants may be part of a heart-protective diet.

MEDIA HYPE

While antioxidants in food are beneficial in many ways, much of what you've likely heard about them is media hype. There is no evidence that supplementation of antioxidants is helpful in reducing the risk of cancer or heart disease, and only moderate evidence that they may be beneficial in fighting aging.

With such hype, the bottom line is this: eating foods rich in antioxidants is healthy and may decrease your risk of disease. However, supplementing antioxidants may actually have negative health consequences. It is important that you discuss your antioxidant status with your doctor, especially if you are considering supplementation.

FOOD SOURCES

It is perfectly safe and even healthy to eat foods high in antioxidants. Blueberries, pomegranates, oranges, carrots, dark leafy greens, and other plant foods are rich in antioxidants and form part of a healthy, disease-preventing diet.

antioxidants

SUPERFOOD: GREEN TEA

Green tea is loaded with antioxidants, which can give you a health boost. It also contains l-theanine, an amino acid that may decrease anxiety and help you relax. Some studies have also shown that green tea may have thermogenic effects: that is, it can increase your metabolism. However, this effect is slight and not what marketers would have you believe. On the other hand, green tea also contains caffeine, which is a stimulant. If you are sensitive to the effects of caffeine, try a decaffeinated version of the tea.

phytonutrients

SUPERFOOD: KALE

Kale seems to be the darling of the nutritional set lately. Is this trendy superfood all it's cracked up to be? While it won't make you instantly young or slim, kale has a lot going for it. It is low in calories and high in fiber. It also contains high levels of vitamins A and C, as well as vitamin B_6, calcium, iron, and magnesium. It's also high in phytonutrients and antioxidants, so it truly is a superstar on your plate.

Phytonutrients, also known as phytochemicals, are compounds derived from plants. While research remains ongoing, many people believe that phytochemicals are responsible for preventing disease. Unlike vitamins and minerals, phytonutrients aren't necessary for survival, but they may help you be healthier. Plant foods contain more than 25,000 different types of phytonutrients. Some are antioxidants, while others may support cell pathways, improve eyesight, or prevent disease. You have probably heard the names of many types of phytonutrients in the news and health talk shows, such as carotenoids, resveratrol, lycopene, and phytoestrogens. Scientists are currently studying the effects these important plant compounds have on the human body.

PHENOLIC ACIDS

Phytochemicals in this class include anthocyanins, flavones, flavanones, and isoflavones. Phenolic acids defend plants against disease and assist in their cell growth. It is believed that when people consume plants high in phenolic acids, these may confer the antioxidant benefits that protect against diseases such as heart disease and certain cancers.

While studies are ongoing into supplementation of phenolic acids such as soy isoflavones and their role in preventing diseases, the results are mixed at best. Ongoing research is still needed. However, consumption of phenolic acids in food may be beneficial to your health. Foods that are high in phenolic acids include:

* Apples
* Artichokes
* Barley
* Berries
* Broccoli
* Buckwheat
* Cabbage
* Celery
* Chiles
* Citrus fruits
* Cocoa
* Kale
* Legumes
* Oats
* Onions
* Peaches
* Potatoes
* Rye
* Soy
* Tomatoes

FLAVONOIDS

Flavonoids are antioxidant compounds in plants with color-providing pigments. In human health, flavonoids may affect cell-signaling pathways as part of a complex system of communication concerning cell activity. They also have significant antioxidant properties.

CANCER

Studies on the effects of flavonoids on cancer have so far not shown that flavonoid consumption reduces the risk of cancer. However, some studies have shown that men with the highest flavonoid consumption had the lowest incidence of developing lung cancer, but in this case the correlation does not indicate causation. More research is required to determine whether it is the flavonoids or some other factor that accounts for this difference.

Other studies have shown inverse correlations between intake of certain flavonoids, such as quercetin and myrecetin, and lung cancer and prostate cancer. In other words, those with higher intake of these two flavonoids had a lower incidence of those diseases. However, more study is required to determine whether the link is causal or merely correlational.

COGNITIVE IMPAIRMENT

There is some evidence suggesting that people who eat higher amounts of flavonoid-containing foods experience lower rates of neurodegenerative disease such as Alzheimer's and Parkinson's diseases but, again, more research is needed. Studies have also shown that diets high in these compounds decrease the risk of developing cognitive impairment, suggesting a protective benefit.

HEART DISEASE

Eating a diet rich in flavonoids appears to have a protective effect against heart disease, but research results are mixed. Some studies show a significant reduction in cardiac risk factors with the intake of flavonoids, while others show a negligible effect. Studies have also shown that dietary flavonoid intake may reduce the risk of stroke, whereas other studies have shown no relationship between the two. The need for ongoing research in this area remains.

SUPERFOOD: CHOCOLATE

Could it be? A dessert that's good for you? It's true that chocolate is an excellent source of flavonoids, and if you're eating chocolate in the form of cocoa powder (perhaps in a fruit smoothie), then it's pretty healthy. However, if you're eating your chocolate in the form of a candy bar, then the sugar, fat, and empty calories are probably having more negative health effects than you're getting from the cocoa. For the best results, choose raw, unprocessed cocoa powder. If you put it in a smoothie, you can sweeten it with a bit of stevia.

Some studies have shown that flavonoids provide a protective benefit in cardiac patients. They appear to help heart disease by facilitating relaxation of the arteries, known as vasodilation, as well as inhibition of platelet aggregation, which can lead to the formations of clots.

FLAVONOID-RICH FOODS

Eating foods rich in flavonoids is part of a healthy, disease-preventing diet. Foods that are high in flavonoids are those with deep colors, and include:

* Apples
* Apricots
* Berries
* Broccoli
* Celery
* Chiles
* Citrus fruits
* Dark chocolate
* Dark leafy greens
* Leeks
* Oregano
* Parsley
* Red cabbage
* Red grapes
* Red wine
* Tea
* Thyme
* Yellow onions

EATING A DIET HIGH IN PHYTONUTRIENTS

Because little benefit has been shown related to supplementation of phytochemicals, it may be a waste of money to take them in supplement form. Eating a diet rich in plant foods in an array of vivid colors can ensure you get the disease-prevention benefits of these healthful compounds without any risks that may be associated with supplementation.

Here are some tips for adopting a diet high in phytonutrients:

* Eat several servings of fruits and vegetables every day.
* Choose 1 cup of food in each of the colors—dark greens, vibrant reds, bright oranges and yellows, purples, and whites—each day.
* Eat plant foods when they are in season, at the peak of ripeness.
* Drink green, black, or white tea.
* Enjoy moderate consumption of dark chocolate and red wine.
* Add fresh herbs to your foods, such as parsley and thyme.
* Add soy to your diet.
* Eat a diet that is varied.

COLORS OF THE RAINBOW

Bright colors indicate high levels of phytonutrients.

Green Green fruits and vegetables contribute phytonutrients such as isoflavones, flavonoids, and lutein. Consider adding the following greens to your meals each day:

* Beet greens
* Broccoli
* Brussels sprouts
* Cabbage
* Collard greens
* Kale
* Mustard greens
* Peas
* Romaine lettuce
* Spinach
* Swiss chard

Red Red fruits and veggies add phytochemicals like lycopene and hydroxybenzoic acid. Adding red to your diet is easy:

* Cherries
* Pomegranate
* Raspberries
* Red cabbage
* Red chiles
* Red grapes
* Strawberries
* Tomatoes

Yellow/Orange Yellow and orange fruits, vegetables, and spices are high in beta-carotene, phthalides, and flavonols:

* Carrots
* Citrus fruits
* Ginger
* Mangos
* Nectarines
* Peaches
* Pineapple
* Pumpkin
* Sweet potatoes
* Turmeric
* Winter squash

White White fruits and vegetables contribute flavonols, quercetin, and allicin:

* Apples
* Coconut
* Garlic
* Onions
* Turnips

SUPERFOOD: SPINACH

With so many ways to prepare it, this dark leafy green is a super-star when it comes to meal planning. Spinach is delicious raw, in salads, or sautéed with a little olive oil and lemon juice. It's also very low in calories and contains a moderate amount of fiber. Spinach is high in vitamin A, vitamin C, iron, potassium, vitamin B_6, and magnesium. Because it is so low in calories and sugars, it's a perfect nutritionally dense food to provide plenty of vitamins and minerals without extra calories.

Blue/Purple These deeply colored fruits and veggies contain anthocyanins and resveratrol, among others:

* Beets
* Blackberries
* Blueberries
* Cocoa
* Eggplant
* Figs
* Purple grapes
* Purple potatoes
* Red wine

Nutrition scientists have long known that eating a diet rich in fruits and vegetables is essential for developing good health and reducing the risk of disease. While some of this is likely attributable to the presence of phytonutrients in fresh fruits and veggies, scientific research remains ongoing. However, whether science eventually bears out the healthfulness of phytonutrients, one fact remains: eating a variety of colorful fruits and vegetables at each meal serves as the foundation of a nutritious, health-promoting diet.

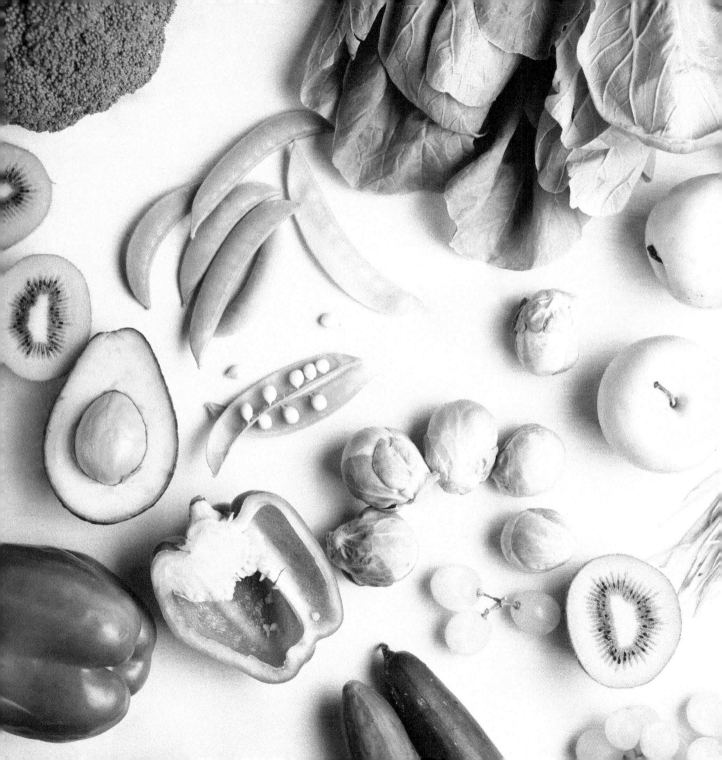

eating

The best way to provide your body with good nutrition is to eat whole foods. Whole foods are those foods that are as close to their natural form as possible. Many of these foods exist around the edges of the supermarket. There, you'll find foods without a lot of added ingredients, such as fresh fruits and vegetables, animal proteins like meat and seafood, and dairy products. When you venture into the inner aisles, avoid the shelves packed with processed foods that tend to contain added sugars, artificial colors and flavors, and similar ingredients. Fill your cart instead with healthy whole grains and legumes like quinoa and rice, as well as fruits and vegetables that have been flash-frozen but don't contain additives. Shopping in this manner allows you to bring home whole foods to nourish your body.

food

The foods you eat are vitally important to your overall health. Choosing a wide variety of unprocessed foods and fresh fruits and vegetables in all kinds of colors will help you get the micro- and macronutrients you need. Understanding food labels and learning something about the nutrients in foods will help you create a healthful diet.

MEAT

For many Americans, meat and poultry serve as the centerpiece for most of their meals. Foods in this category include chicken, turkey, duck, beef, lamb, pork, game meats, and organ meats.

MEAT NUTRITION

Nutritionally, meat and poultry consist of protein and fat, and also contain vitamins and minerals.

Meat and poultry offer an excellent source of complete protein. They are also a strong source of essential vitamins and minerals, including iron, vitamins B_6 and B_{12}, niacin, thiamin, riboflavin, vitamin E, magnesium, and zinc.

The fat in meat is mostly saturated fat. However, it does contain moderate amounts of polyunsaturated fatty acids (PUFAs) as well, which may provide protective benefits against heart disease.

Organ meats (offal), such as liver, kidneys, and heart—once commonplace on American dinner plates—are working their way back into American kitchens thanks to their nutritional density. Organ meats are especially high in iron, vitamin A, vitamins B_2 and B_{12}, zinc, and folate.

MEAT LABELING

In supermarkets in the United States, you'll find several different labels on meat that indicate how the meat was raised and designate the quality of the meat you are purchasing. The USDA controls how manufacturers can label their meat.

GRAIN-FED BEEF

The majority of beef and dairy cattle in the United States are fed grain, primarily corn. This is because corn is a cheap source of feed, and it fattens the cattle quickly. Grain-fed beef tends to be fattier than grass-fed. In general, these cattle are raised in factory farming operations that house thousands of cattle in small pens. Due to the packed real estate these cows inhabit, they often stand, sit, and sleep in feces. Disease can spread easily among factory-farmed cattle, which may make it more likely for this type of beef to bear foodborne pathogens.

- **Certified:** Certified meats have been evaluated by USDA inspectors to certify that the way the meat is labeled meets their standards.
- **Free Range/Free Roaming:** These labels on poultry mean that the birds have access to the outdoors. Neither label, however, sets standards for how much space the birds have to roam, how much time birds spend outside, their outdoor and indoor living conditions, or similar considerations.
- **Natural:** Meat labeled "natural" has been minimally processed and contains no artificial ingredients.
- **No Hormones:** Federal law prohibits the use of hormones with hogs and fowl, so this label does not appear on pork or poultry products. The same prohibition, however, is not applied to cattle, so be sure to look for the "no hormones" label to choose beef products that come from cattle raised without hormones.
- **No Antibiotics:** This label indicates that poultry and beef products come from animals raised without the use of antibiotics.
- **Organic:** An "organic" label means that the animals were raised in a way that meets federal organic standards, typically with only organic feed and without the use of antibiotics or hormones.

GRASS-FED VERSUS GRAIN-FED

In the United States, there has been a growing interest in meat from pastured or grass-fed animals versus grain-fed animals. There is a difference in taste, texture, and fat profiles between the two types of meats.

"Grass-fed" is a label you'll primarily see with beef, buffalo, and bison meat. Grass-fed cattle are raised spending time feeding on grass in pastures, as opposed to eating grain in factory farming operations. Grass-fed meats tend to have less total fat than their grain-fed counterparts, and they are also higher in omega-3 fatty acids, conjugated linoleic acid (CLA), and antioxidant vitamins.

GRASS-FED BEEF

Grass-fed beef has been showing up a lot recently in supermarket meat departments. Grass-fed beef comes from cattle that have been allowed to graze naturally on pasturelands instead of being fed grains. Grass-fed beef tends to be leaner than grain-fed, and also higher in omega-3 fatty acids and conjugated linoleic acid. Because the cattle feed on grass, the beef is also higher in a number of vitamins and minerals, such as vitamin E and beta-carotene.

ORGANIC

In the United States, the USDA controls labeling of organic foods. Foods labeled "organic" must meet rigorous standards. In general, organic foods may not be genetically modified, and may not be grown with pesticides. Organic meat must not have hormones or antibiotics included in the animals' feed. Only foods that contain all-organic ingredients can carry the label "100 percent organic." Other organic labels may say, "Contains organic ingredients." In this case, it is likely that only some of the ingredients are organic.

LEANEST CUTS OF MEAT AND POULTRY

People watching their weight may wish to select cuts of meat that are lower in fat in order to reduce caloric intake. While current research suggests that dietary intake of saturated fat and cholesterol is not as unhealthy as previously believed, fat is more calorically dense (it has 9 calories per gram versus 4 calories per gram in protein). Therefore, meats with higher levels of fat will have more calories. If you're watching calories, choose leaner meats and poultry, such as boneless, skinless chicken or turkey breast, pork tenderloin, beef tenderloin, and beef strip steak. To make the meat even leaner, trim all visible fat.

RECOMMENDATIONS

The US Dietary Guideline Committee's 2015 report makes recommendations for daily protein consumption. The report points out that while animal proteins can be used to meet these recommendations, the protein can come from plant sources, too. The report recommends reducing or minimizing meat and poultry consumption and replacing it with seafood or plant sources of protein.

DAIRY

Dairy products include milk, yogurt, cheese, cream, butter, and other items that come from cows, goats, or sheep. Calcium-fortified soymilk also fits in this group.

DAIRY NUTRITION

The Dairy Council has done an excellent job of getting the message out about one of dairy's key nutrients: calcium. Dairy products are much more than calcium, however.

* **Carbohydrates:** Dairy products vary in carbohydrate levels. In general, in dairy without added sugar, the more fat the dairy product has per serving, the fewer carbs it has. Carbohydrates in dairy products come from lactose, which is a simple sugar. This sugar is naturally present in milk products.
* **Protein:** Dairy products contain a moderate amount of protein, which varies according to the product. One cup of 1% milk

has about 8 grams of protein, which is around 3 percent by volume.

Milk contains two primary proteins: casein and whey. In cow's milk, casein makes up about 80 percent of the milk's protein content, and it is the primary protein in hard cheeses. The remaining 20 percent of protein in cow's milk dairy products is whey, which is used to make soft and curdled cheeses such as cottage cheese or ricotta.

* **Fat:** The fat profile in dairy products is a combination of saturated and unsaturated fats, with the majority (around 75 percent) coming from saturated fat. The types of unsaturated fats and the fatty acid profile of the dairy products depend largely on the way the dairy cattle are raised, as well as on whether they are grass- or grain-fed.

  Fat content varies greatly, with low-fat and skim milk products having the lowest amount of fat, and full-fat milk, cream, cheese, and butter having the highest.

* **Micronutrients:** Milk contains a number of essential micronutrients. The best-known of these is calcium. Some milk is fortified with vitamin D to enhance calcium absorption. Milk is also high in potassium and contains phosphorus, zinc, magnesium, and vitamin B_{12}.

FREE-RANGE

Free-range is a term used in poultry labeling. For poultry or eggs to be labeled free-range, the animals must have access to the outdoors, such as a door they can go out through. This doesn't mean, however, that the poultry ever actually makes it outdoors—oftentimes "free range" poultry stays put in a crowded henhouse.

RAW MILK

Milk that comes fresh from the cow and undergoes no processing is known as "raw milk." You can find dairy products made from raw milk in natural foods and grocery stores, although the FDA warns that it may harbor microorganisms, such as *E. coli* or salmonella, which pose a threat to health.

PASTEURIZATION AND HOMOGENIZATION

Because of the threat of foodborne illness from raw milk consumption, most dairy producers pasteurize milk, which involves heating it to a certain temperature and keeping it there for a specific period. This procedure kills the potentially harmful bacteria in the milk. According to the FDA, the process does nothing to affect the milk's nutritional content.

To keep the milk from separating into liquids and fats, producers also homogenize the milk, using a mechanical process to break down the fat solids so they mix in with the liquids and do not separate.

DAIRY LABELING

Like meat, the FDA controls the claims made on dairy labels.

* **Skim/Nonfat, 1%, 2%, Whole Milk:** Labels on milk will tell you the fat content by volume (not by calories) of fat in the milk. Skim/nonfat milk has less than 1 percent fat by volume. Whole milk contains both the milk and the cream, and with no attempt to reduce the fat in the milk.
* **Natural:** While the term "natural" isn't specifically defined in FDA rules, the label indicates that no artificial ingredients have been added to the product.
* **Organic:** This indicates that the dairy cattle have been raised following organic standards, which typically means the cattle have been fed organic feed and given no hormones or antibiotics.

GRASS-FED VERSUS GRAIN-FED

In the same manner that cattle raised for meat can be raised either eating grass or grains, so can dairy cows—and with similar benefits.

RECOMMENDATIONS

The USDA's MyPlate recommendations suggest the following dairy intake by age:

* 2 to 3 years: 2 cups daily
* 4 to 8 years: 2½ cups daily
* 9 years and older: 3 cups daily

In these guidelines, 1 cup of milk, yogurt, or soymilk is equivalent to 1½ ounces of natural cheese or 2 ounces of processed cheese.

food

SEAFOOD

Fish and shellfish are a delicious and healthy part of a balanced diet. Foods in this category include freshwater fish, such as trout and catfish; ocean fish, such as halibut and salmon; and shellfish, such as shrimp, clams, and oysters.

SEAFOOD NUTRITION

Seafood is an excellent source of lean protein. While fish and shellfish do contain fat, the content tends to be low and mostly unsaturated. Because of this low level of fat, fish tends to be lower in calories than other types of animal proteins. Fish also contains a number of vital micronutrients.

* **Protein:** Protein in fish and shellfish ranges from 16 to 26 grams per 3-ounce serving. Because of the ratio of high protein to low fat, many people who are trying to cut back on calories and fat may prefer fish as their primary animal protein.
* **Fat:** A 3-ounce serving of fish and seafood contains 0.5 to 10 grams of fat per serving. That's an extremely low-fat form of animal protein. Fish and shellfish that have the most fat include salmon, trout, mackerel, catfish, and oysters.

  While a small amount of the fat in some types of fish and shellfish (such as trout, oysters, salmon, perch, catfish, and tilapia) is saturated, fish is also an excellent source of PUFAs as well as beneficial omega-3 fatty acids. In fact, fish is the best dietary source of these essential omega-3 fatty acids. Fish highest in EFAs include wild-caught salmon, anchovies, mackerel, sablefish, whitefish, sardines, tuna, herring, and trout.
* **Micronutrients:** Seafood contains a number of essential vitamins and minerals, including B-complex vitamins, vitamin A, vitamin D, iodine, selenium, iron, and zinc.

MERCURY AND SEAFOOD

All fish and shellfish contain traces of mercury, which come from mercury concentrations in the ocean. In most cases, the amount is so small that it is not a problem. However, consumption of mercury in larger amounts, especially by children or pregnant women, may lead to nervous system

WILD-CAUGHT FISH AND SEAFOOD

Wild-caught seafood comes from the ocean, where it swims freely in its natural habitat until fishermen catch it. Fish and seafood that swim freely in the ocean eat foods that they are meant to eat, such as algae, plankton, sea vegetables, and other fish. The food the fish eats, as well as the activity of swimming freely in the ocean, affect its nutrient levels, rendering it high in omega-3 fatty acids. Wild-caught seafood tends to be relatively free of contaminants.

FARMED FISH AND SHELLFISH

Farmed fish and shellfish are farmed in saltwater pens with lots of other sea animals. The crowded conditions in these pens allow disease to spread easily. A 2004 study showed that farmed seafood was much higher in PCBs, a potentially harmful chemical, than wild-caught seafood. There are contradictory studies about whether farmed fish and shellfish have the same nutrition levels as wild-caught fish and shellfish. Often, however, farmed fish are fed diets that the species doesn't typically eat, such as corn or soy. This can change the nutritional profile of the seafood.

damage. Therefore, it is important to avoid fish and shellfish that contain high levels of mercury. Choosing fish with only trace amounts can help you enjoy the health benefits of fish consumption without the dangers associated with high mercury intake.

You should avoid eating the following fish, which have the highest levels of mercury: king mackerel, marlin, orange roughy, shark, swordfish, tilefish, and bigeye tuna. Fish with relatively high mercury levels, such as bluefish, grouper, mackerel, Chilean sea bass, albacore tuna, and yellowfin tuna, can be consumed up to three times per month.

You can regularly enjoy fish and shellfish in the following category; these have the least amount of mercury: anchovies, calamari, catfish, clams, crab, flounder, haddock, herring, oyster, perch, pollock, salmon, sardines, scallops, shrimp, sole, tilapia, trout, and whitefish.

FISH LABELING

The FDA has established a few labeling regulations, including labeling seafood with its country of origin. (Processed seafood is exempt from this law.) Some fish may have an organic label, but there are currently no labeling standards for designating seafood as organic.

WILD-CAUGHT VERSUS FARMED

One label you may see on fish and seafood is either "wild-caught" or "farm raised." Wild-caught fish are those caught by fishermen in their natural habitats: oceans, rivers, bays, and lakes. Farmed or farm-raised fish and shellfish are cultivated in seafood "farms." The open-water swimming of wild-caught seafood lowers fat levels and produces a higher concentration of healthy omega-3 fatty acids. Farmed fish may also be more susceptible to disease, and they may contain higher levels of contaminants from pollution that collects in the pens where the seafood is raised.

RECOMMENDATIONS

The 2015 Dietary Guidelines Advisory Committee report recommends that Americans eat three to six servings of seafood per week. A serving of fish is 3 to 4 ounces. Choose fish that is low in mercury but high in omega-3 fatty acids.

VEGETABLES

According to the 2015 Dietary Guidelines for Americans, people should aim to make vegetables the largest portion of their diet. Vegetables are highly nutritious and naturally low in fats and calories, and contain fiber.

LEAFY GREENS

Leafy greens include vegetables such as spinach, kale, chard, arugula, and lettuce. They contain fiber and are very low in simple sugars. They are also packed with nutrition, with many such as kale and spinach classified as superfoods. In leafy greens, you'll find hefty amounts of vitamins A, C, and K, as well as folic acid, iron, antioxidants, and phytochemicals. They also fill you up while being extremely low in calories thanks to their negligible fat content.

ROOT VEGETABLES/TUBERS

Root vegetables and tubers are those vegetables that grow underground. Vegetables in this category include onions, turnips, carrots, parsnips, rutabaga, sweet potatoes, radishes, and celeriac. Root vegetables tend to have moderate levels of starch and carbohydrates, but they also contain plenty of fiber. Root vegetables also contain vitamins C and A, folic acid, potassium, and manganese.

STALK VEGETABLES

Stalk vegetables include asparagus, fennel, celery, and rhubarb. Stalk vegetables are usually very high in fiber and very low in calories, and they contain vitamins and minerals.

CRUCIFEROUS VEGETABLES

Cruciferous vegetables include veggies like cabbage, broccoli, cauliflower, and Brussels sprouts. These vegetables are low in calories and high in fiber, and they contain lots of antioxidants like vitamins C, E, and K. They also contain folate and trace minerals.

NIGHTSHADES

The nightshade family comprises bell peppers, potatoes, tomatoes, and eggplant. Many of these vegetables are brightly colored. Colorful vegetables generally contain larger amounts of nutrients, including vitamins C

food

GMO

GMO stands for genetically modified organism. GMOs have been altered using bioengineering techniques. Genetic modification occurs for many reasons, such as increasing crop yields or conferring pest resistance. Little research exists into the long-term health effects of consuming genetically modified foods. Currently, there are no federal labeling laws requiring food manufacturers to let you know when food contains GMOs. It is estimated that about 70 percent of processed foods contain at least one GMO ingredient.

and A and the antioxidant lycopene. They are low in calories and also contain fiber.

Nightshades contain alkaloids, to which some people react with muscle pain and other health issues. People sensitive to nightshades should avoid them.

GREEN BEANS

While technically a member of the legume family, green beans are eaten as a vegetable and packed with tasty nutrition. They are low in calories and high in fiber, and they contain vitamins C and K, folate, manganese, magnesium, and a number of other vitamins and minerals.

SQUASH

Squash refers to both summer and winter squash. Pumpkin, butternut squash, acorn squash, zucchini, and pattypan squash are all members of the squash family. Squash is low in calories and high in water and fiber. Summer squash (zucchini-type squash) contains vitamin C, copper, manganese, magnesium, phosphorus, and potassium, while winter squash contains vitamins A, B_6, and C, plus manganese and copper.

MUSHROOMS

Mushrooms are technically a fungus, although many people consume them as a vegetable. They are very low in calories and contain high levels of vitamin B_2 and B_3, copper, selenium, pantothenic acid, and phosphorus.

SEA VEGETABLES

Sea vegetables don't show up on the plate of many Americans, but they pack a powerful nutritional punch. Sea vegetables include foods such as dulse, kelp, and wakame. They are high in vitamin C, iron, iodine, and manganese.

ORGANIC VERSUS CONVENTIONALLY GROWN

Conventionally grown vegetables may have trace residue of pesticides from the farming process. Organically grown vegetables are farmed without these pesticides. The Environmental Working Group regularly publishes a list called the Dirty Dozen and the Clean Fifteen that shows which vegetables contain the highest amounts of pesticide residue and should therefore be purchased organic, as well as those that have minimal residue and can be purchased as conventionally grown. The current dirty dozen includes celery, spinach, bell peppers, cucumbers, cherry tomatoes, kale, snap peas, collard greens, and hot peppers. The clean fifteen includes avocadoes, cabbage, onions, asparagus, eggplant, cauliflower, and sweet potatoes.

RECOMMENDATIONS

According to MyPlate, vegetable recommendations vary by age group and by the type of vegetable. In general, the FDA recommends eating a variety of vegetables, including dark leafy greens, red and orange vegetables, beans and peas, starchy vegetables, and others. Children need as much as 18 cups of vegetables per week, while adults need as much as 21 cups per week.

FRUITS

Fruits are foods that come from trees and contain seeds. There are a number of different types of fruits that confer various health benefits.

CITRUS FRUITS

Citrus fruits are juicy, flavorful fruits with a thick peel. They include oranges, grapefruit, lemons, limes, and tangerines. They are high in flavonoids, as well as antioxidants such as vitamin C, folate, and B-complex vitamins.

Citrus fruits have moderate levels of fructose, and they contain some fiber. Eating the whole fruit helps you limit the sugar consumption, while juicing increases the proportion of sugar and calories in each serving.

TREE FRUITS

Tree fruits, like apples, pears, and figs, are fall-harvested fruits with an edible outer peel. Apples have moderate calories and fiber. They also contain a moderate amount of fructose, which is a simple sugar. They contain vitamin A and vitamin B_6. Pears have a similar nutritional profile to apples, although they tend to be slightly sweeter and thus slightly higher in sugar. Figs are high in fiber and fructose. They contain vitamin B_6.

STONE FRUITS

Stone fruits are those that contain a pit in the middle. They include peaches, plums, nectarines, cherries, and apricots. Stone fruits contain moderate levels of calories, fructose, and fiber. They are high in vitamins A and C, as well as phytonutrients and antioxidants.

BERRIES

Berries are high in fiber and have relatively low levels of fructose. They are also low in calories. Because of their deep coloring, berries are high in antioxidants and phytochemicals.

MELONS

Melons have a high water and fiber content, combined with a low fructose concentration. They tend to be relatively low in calories. They are also high in potassium and vitamins A, C, and B_6 and contain a small amount of iron.

TROPICAL FRUITS

Tropical fruits include bananas, papayas, passion fruit, guavas, pineapples, and mangos. These fruits tend to be high in fructose and therefore more calorically dense than other fruits. These juicy fruits are high in potassium, vitamin C, phytonutrients, and enzymes.

DRIED FRUITS

Dried fruits, such as apples, raisins, and dates, contain a concentration of nutrients. Because the water has been evaporated, they also tend to be quite high in fructose and calories per volume. After drying, they still retain the micronutrient properties of their fresh counterparts.

GRAPES

Grapes are high in water and vitamin K. They contain moderate amounts of fructose and fiber, and they are relatively low-calorie. Dark-skinned grapes contain high levels of flavonols, carotenoids, and phenolic acids, which are antioxidants.

FRESH, CANNED, OR FROZEN?

You can buy fruits (and vegetables) in fresh, canned, or frozen form. Fresh fruits tend to maintain their nutrient content the best and have the best flavor, but flash-frozen fruits are a close second. Frozen fruits make a great backup plan when fresh fruits aren't in season. If you choose canned fruit, pick those without additives and those that are packed in water and not a sugar syrup.

ORGANIC VERSUS CONVENTIONAL

According to the Environmental Working Group, the following fruits should be purchased organically grown because they contain high levels of pesticides: apples, peaches, nectarines, strawberries, and grapes. Fruit you can purchase conventionally grown (because they contain minimal traces of pesticide) include avocados, pineapples, mangos, kiwis, grapefruit, and cantaloupe.

RECOMMENDATIONS

Daily fruit recommendations vary depending on age, sex, and activity level. Because of their nutrient content, you do need to include some fruit in your diet every day.

Note that people with higher activity levels may require more fruit in their daily diet.

RDA: FRUIT

The MyPlate daily fruit recommendations are as follows:

Boys, 2 to 18 years	1 to 2 cups
Girls, 2 to 18 years	1 to 1½ cups
Men, over 18 years	2 cups
Women, 19 to 30 years	2 cups
Women, over 30 years	1½ cups

drink

Often, when people think about eating, they don't account for the beverages they include with their meals and throughout the day. However, what you drink can be as vitally important to your health as what you eat. Drinking cola or other types of soda adds sugar and empty calories to your daily intake. Juice adds nutrients but also increases sugar and calories. Alcohol changes the order in which you process energy, but it also has some health benefits. Coffee and tea contain caffeine, but may also confer health benefits. All beverages contain water, which is essential to good health, but how do the beverages you consume fit in with your overall nutritional plan?

COFFEE AND TEA

Coffee and tea continue to surge in popularity in the United States. Coffee shops seem to be popping up both on and between nearly every street corner in every city, and many people feel they can't make it through the day without their cup of coffee or tea.

CAFFEINE

The substance in your coffee and tea that provides your get-up-and-go is caffeine. That's because caffeine is a stimulant, which can have various effects including serving as a diuretic and blunting appetite.

Caffeine is also a drug that is used daily by about 80 percent of the American adult population. Caffeine affects the body by working as a central nervous system stimulant. While it can increase alertness, it may have side effects such as a rise in blood pressure, rapid heartbeat, jitteriness, headaches, and dehydration. Caffeine may cause additional issues in people with heart disease, and it may exacerbate symptoms in people who experience anxiety.

This stimulant is physically and psychologically addictive. Suddenly ceasing consumption can create symptoms of withdrawal, including irritability, flu-like symptoms, lethargy, and headaches. Withdrawal symptoms can last for as long as a week, which can be uncomfortable but is not life-threatening.

Caffeine can help improve alertness and concentration for short periods. It also works as an antioxidant, speeds up metabolism, dampens appetite for weight loss, and can help relieve migraine headaches by dilating blood vessels in the head.

HEALTH BENEFITS OF COFFEE

Fortunately, if you're one of the millions of Americans addicted to your daily cup of joe, it could be conferring some health benefits as well:

* Some studies, including an 11-year study published in 2006 in the *Archives of Internal Medicine*, showed that coffee consumption seemed to provide protective benefits against the development of type 2 diabetes.
* Multiple studies have shown that coffee may have protective benefits against liver disease, and regular consumption may provide relief of certain symptoms associated with liver disease.
* Coffee is high in antioxidants, which can protect the body against and remove signs of oxidative stress caused by free radicals.
* A 2012 study showed that coffee consumption may help patients with Parkinson's disease achieve better motor control.
* By itself, coffee is low in calories.

HEALTH BENEFITS OF TEA

Not all tea contains caffeine. Herbal teas are free from caffeine, and some green and black teas are conventionally decaffeinated. Like coffee, research indicates that tea may confer health benefits to regular drinkers.

* Tea contains polyphenols, which provide protective benefits against heart disease.
* Tea also contains flavonoids, including EGCG, which protect against clogged arteries and certain cancers.

* Green tea may help improve cholesterol and reduce the risk of developing neurological disorders because it contains high concentrations of EGCG.
* Herbal teas may have medicinal properties. Chamomile tea is well-known for promoting relaxation and sleep, while echinacea tea may boost the immune system to help you fight off colds.

KEEPING COFFEE AND TEA HEALTHY

The best way to reap the benefits of coffee and tea without experiencing the drawbacks is to consume them in moderation (one or two cups per day). How you take your coffee or tea also has a lot to do with how it affects you.

* **Drink It Black:** Drink your coffee or tea black. If you must have it sweetened, choose a natural, noncaloric sweetener like stevia. Adding sugar increases the calorie count of the beverages, which can spike blood sugar and cause weight gain. Avoid artificial sweeteners.

    If you like your coffee or tea "light," try adding skim milk, almond milk, coconut milk, or soymilk instead of cream, which is high in saturated fat and calories. Avoid nondairy creamers, which are high in trans and saturated fats and often contain sugar.
* **Skip the Fussy Drinks:** A daily double venti mochaccino with extra whipped cream and a shot of syrup adds a lot of empty calories to your diet. That can lead to weight gain. Less calorie-loaded alternatives include an Americano, which contains espresso and water, or a "skinny" latte made with either skim milk or a low-fat dairy substitute such as soymilk or rice milk.

ALCOHOL

Whether you enjoy a glass of red wine with dinner, sip a beer on a hot afternoon, or slam shots of hard liquor with your friends on the weekends, alcohol has a definite effect on your health.

DEPENDENCE

Alcohol is a physically and psychologically addictive substance. Regularly consuming alcohol can lead to increased alcohol tolerance and even addiction. You may lose control, neglect important activities in your life, or experience physical effects of the alcohol.

If you become addicted to alcohol, you may have difficulty stopping. Withdrawing from alcohol may require medical supervision because of potentially severe withdrawal symtoms such as delirium tremens, agitation, fevers, hallucinations, seizures, and confusion.

ALCOHOL METABOLISM

The body rids itself of a small percentage of consumed alcohol via sweat and urination. The majority, however, remains in the body and must be metabolized. Because your body needs to lower your blood concentrations of alcohol as quickly as possible, it metabolizes the alcohol first, before metabolizing any other food or drink. This is significant if you are trying to lose weight, because your body will always burn alcohol before it burns any additional calories or stored fat.

The majority of alcohol metabolism occurs in the liver. This can lead to scarring in the liver. Over the long term, it can lead to a condition called cirrhosis.

NEGATIVE HEALTH EFFECTS

Long-term heavy use of alcohol may lead to a host of health effects, including anemia, certain cancers, cirrhosis of the liver (liver scarring), dementia, nerve damage, and other health problems.

* **Dehydration:** Alcohol is a diuretic, which causes your body to excrete water. Heavy alcohol consumption can lead to dehydration.
* **Weight Gain:** As previously mentioned, alcohol may stop your body from using its fat stores for fuel, which may prevent weight loss or even lead to weight gain. How you drink your alcohol may also contribute additional calories that can make weight more difficult to manage.

drink

ALCOHOL CALORIC CONTENT

Alcohol has 7 calories per gram, which is higher than the 4 per gram in carbs and protein and less than the 9 calories per gram in fat. Your body always metabolizes alcohol before it metabolizes other macronutrients, however, so if you're trying to lose weight, alcohol consumption can hamper weight loss. Many alcoholic beverages get their caloric content from both the alcohol and whatever it is mixed with. Dry wines, liquors, and light beer have the lowest caloric content among drinks, but beware of mixers adding calories to your drinks.

Alcohol itself has 7 calories per gram, which is fewer calories per gram than fat but more than carbs and proteins. What may contribute even more to weight gain than the alcohol itself is the form in which you drink it. Dry wines and light beers are relatively low in calories. Drinking sweet wines, beer, or drinks with sugary or creamy mixers may add empty calories to your diet.

* **Folate Absorption:** The Harvard T. H. Chan School of Public Health notes that alcohol consumption blocks absorption of the B vitamin folate, which is important for human growth and development. Supplementing folate or eating foods that contain it can help minimize this issue.

* **Breast Cancer:** Several studies show that alcohol consumption can increase the risk of developing breast cancer. Having two or more drinks per day may increase risk by as much as 41 percent.

* **Fetal Development:** Pregnant women who consume alcohol regularly may risk causing harm to their infants. The alcohol enters the mother's bloodstream and travels into the baby's developing organs. Because the baby doesn't break down alcohol as quickly as an adult, it remains in his or her body for much longer. This can lead to a condition in infants called fetal alcohol syndrome. The effects of fetal alcohol syndrome can last a lifetime, and may include low birth weight, behavioral or attention problems, defects of the heart, slowed growth, poor muscle tone, and learning difficulties.

HEALTH BENEFITS

Moderate intake (one to two drinks per day) of alcohol may confer health benefits. According to the Harvard T. H. Chan School of Public Health, moderate consumption of alcohol may lower the risk of developing cardiovascular disease.

A 1985 national health survey showed that people who reported moderate drinking were more likely to be of normal weight than those who didn't drink at all or drank heavily. Moderate drinkers reported exercising regularly and having healthy sleep habits. Moderate drinkers were also less likely to develop type 2 diabetes and gallstones.

JUICES

Most people consider juice a healthy substance, and certainly there's a lot to recommend it. Juice comes from fresh fruits and vegetables, and it contains the same phytonutrients, vitamins, and minerals that the fruits and vegetables contain. What it lacks, however, is the fiber, and this makes it less filling than eating a whole piece of fruit or vegetable.

BENEFITS OF JUICE

Juice confers many of the same health benefits you get from the fruit or vegetable from which the juice was obtained. The healthiest form of juice is freshly squeezed juice, which is high in vitamins, minerals, and phytochemicals. These nutrients can provide protective benefits against heart disease, cancer, and other illnesses while fighting oxidative stress caused by free radicals.

For people who don't like fresh fruits and vegetables or find them difficult to eat, juicing is a flavorful way to get the health benefits without having to eat the whole fruit or veggie. Fruit juice also serves as a healthier stand-in for sugar in baked goods and desserts.

IS JUICING HEALTHIER THAN EATING FRUITS OF VEGETABLES?

According to the Mayo Clinic, juicing isn't healthier than eating the fruit or vegetable whole. While some people believe that juicing makes the nutrients in fruits and vegetables more readily available to the body, no evidence exists that this is so.

FRUCTOSE

One of the biggest issues with fruit juice is its sugar content. When you eat a whole piece of fruit, you get a little bit of fruit sugar that is mixed in with the fiber in the plant. While fruit does contain small amounts of fructose, eating it in solid fruit form helps keep blood sugar steady and doesn't cause harm to your body.

However, when you juice fruit, several things happen. First, the fiber is removed from the fruit, so your body will burn the sugar in the fruit much more quickly. It also takes a lot more than a single piece of fruit to provide a serving of juice. This means that you are getting the calories and sugar

drink

PRESSED JUICE

Cold-pressed juices are created by pressing fresh fruit or vegetables under very high pressure. This pressure renders the juices shelf-stable while maintaining the nutrient profiles of the fresh fruit. Pressed juice also tastes more like freshly squeezed juice than pasteurized juice, so it is considered a premium juice. Because they don't have any additives, preservatives, or added sugar, pressed juices remain relatively healthy. However, juice is still primarily sugar and should be consumed in moderation in a healthy diet.

of several pieces of fruit in an 8-ounce cup of juice, making the juice very calorically dense.

* **In the Liver:** The primary sugar in fruit juice is fructose, which is processed in the body by the liver. According to the Harvard T. H. Chan School of Public Health, the body uses fructose to create fat through a process called lipogenesis. While much of this fat is stored in fat cells, small fat droplets begin to collect in the liver as well. Over time, this can lead to a condition called fatty liver disease. While nonalcoholic fatty liver disease usually remains asymptomatic, in some people it can cause inflammation, which in turn causes scarring, and eventually cirrhosis.

* **In Other Systems:** Excess fructose consumption can cause changes in your body that may increase markers of heart disease. The effects of excessive fructose consumption include increases in triglycerides and low-density lipoproteins (LDL, or "bad" cholesterol), fat buildup around organs, increased blood pressure, and increase of insulin resistance in tissues.

COMMERCIALLY PREPARED JUICES

Commercially prepared juices may contain additives or preservatives, and many also contain added sugars. If you do drink commercially prepared juice, read ingredient labels carefully and look for "100 percent juice" on the label, which indicates that there are no added sugars or preservatives.

JUICE AND DENTAL HEALTH

While drinking 100 percent juice doesn't serve as a threat to the dental health of adults, it can affect the dental health of infants and toddlers consuming it in a bottle. Giving a baby or toddler a bottle of juice can lead to a condition called baby bottle tooth decay. This may occur because the sugars in the juice remain in the mouth and attract cavity-causing bacteria. To prevent this, provide only water, breast milk, or formula in your baby's bottle, and practice regular dental hygiene.

---

drink

PASTEURIZED JUICE

Pasteurized juices are heated in order to kill foodborne pathogens. While this makes the juices stable and safe, it may kill some of the vitamins more susceptible to heat degradation, such as vitamin C. Other nutrients, such as minerals and more stable vitamins, will remain, so the juice is still nutritious. Although they are pasteurized, you still need to refrigerate or freeze these juices to prevent spoilage and discourage the growth of foodborne bacteria.

diets

Millions of Americans are seeking a way to lose weight, and many of them have tried at least one diet. With so much contradictory information available about weight loss, it's difficult to know which diets work, which are sustainable, and which may pose threats to your overall health. In the sections that follow, you'll find information about some of today's most popular diets.

Each of these diets is given a rating from 1 to 10 for weight loss and nutrition, with a score of 10 as the highest rating. Weight loss ratings take into account the effectiveness of each diet as reported in findings of medical studies, and the apparent ease of following the plan and maintenance. For example, a diet that allows 2 or more pounds of weight loss per week, keeps you satiated, and is easy to maintain over time will likely have a higher health rating than a diet where studies show limited weight loss and feelings of hunger. Nutrition ratings take into account the types of foods allowed on the diet and how they relate to the USDA-issued Dietary Guidelines for Americans. A diet that allows for a lot of processed foods and sugar may have a lower health rating, while one with more nutritionally dense, unprocessed foods will have a higher one.

ATKINS DIET

The Atkins diet has been around since 1972, when Dr. Robert Atkins first released his book *Dr. Atkins' Diet Revolution*. Atkins, a cardiologist, developed the diet after losing weight on the basis of information he found in one of his medical journals. Since then, the diet has gone through several refinements. Today's Atkins diet is much less strict than the original Atkins plan, and now includes a number of low-carbohydrate foods such as baking mix, protein bars, shakes, and candy that Atkins Nutritionals sells to complement the diet.

HUNGER

While people use the terms hunger and appetite interchangeably, these terms actually mean very different things. Hunger is the physical need for food. It is biologically driven. Hormones such as ghrelin and leptin control hunger and satiation. Ghrelin increases hunger, while leptin decreases it. Imbalances in these two hormones may cause hunger even when there isn't a biological need for food, or they may cause you to not feel hungry even when you haven't eaten.

APPETITE

Appetite is the mental desire for food. It may have emotional or rational origins. Learning to distinguish appetite from hunger is essential for weight maintenance.

THE BASICS

The Atkins diet is a low-carbohydrate diet. The diet has four phases. In the first phase, Induction, dieters must eat 20 grams or fewer of carbohydrates daily, mostly from nonstarchy vegetables. In the Ongoing Weight Loss (OWL) phase, dieters gradually increase their daily carb intake until they reach a level where they find a sustainable rate of loss. During OWL, dieters may add starchier vegetables like carrots, as well as nuts and seeds. In the current iteration of the diet, people may also add Atkins shakes and other products in this level. In the premaintenance and maintenance phrases, dieters gradually ramp up their carbohydrate intake until they find their individual carbohydrate tolerance level, which will allow them to maintain the weight they have lost.

THE CLAIMS/BENEFITS

The main reason people go on the Atkins diet is to lose weight. According to Atkins Nutritionals, as well as the late Dr. Atkins himself, the diet has other health benefits also, including:

* Reduction of acid reflux and GERD symptoms (see p. 164)
* Reduction of skin breakouts
* Improvement of cardiac risk factors such as cholesterol levels, high blood pressure, and triglycerides
* Improvement of general health

NUTRITIONAL VALUE

The Atkins diet is high in protein and fat and very low in carbohydrates. It is high in vegetables, animal proteins, and saturated fat. Depending on the amount and type of vegetables eaten, it tends to contain low to moderate levels of fiber. If you eat a variety of vegetables and avoid eating processed foods—including those offered by Atkins Nutritionals—then the diet is very nutrient-dense.

SHORT-TERM EFFECTS

Anecdotal evidence suggests that the Atkins diet is very effective in the short term. Atkins dieters tout weight loss in the first two weeks of the diet of as much as 15 pounds.

Research into the Atkins diet shows short-term health effects, including:

- An increased rate of weight loss as compared to low-fat and calorie-restricted diets in the first three months
- Improved HDL cholesterol
- Loss of excess water weight

During the first week, dieters on Atkins may notice several symptoms that will go away after the first few days. Referred to as "Atkins flu," dieters may notice flu-like symptoms such as lethargy and fatigue. As the body makes the switch to burning ketones, however, many dieters notice improved energy levels and better sleep.

LONG-TERM EFFECTS

The Atkins diet does promote long-term weight loss, but the weight loss is maintained only if the dieter follows the plan and makes permanent lifestyle changes. If the dieter returns to eating carbohydrates, the lost weight will return.

Research shows other long-term health effects of Atkins, including:

- Sustained weight loss if the dieter continues restricting carbohydrates
- Lowered risk of developing type 2 diabetes
- Lowered LDL and triglyceride levels

HEALTH AND WEIGHT LOSS RATING

The Atkins diet has much to recommend it, but there are also concerns.

Pros:

- The diet is high in whole foods—if one avoids the processed Atkins Nutritionals products.
- It contains plenty of vegetables.
- It contains adequate protein.
- Quick weight loss is motivating.
- If followed properly, the diet promotes sustained weight loss.

CLIMATE AND NUTRITION

Climate change has a significant impact on nutrition. As temperatures and weather patterns change in regions around the world, the types of crops that can be grown there may change accordingly. Climate change also affects the quality of the air, soil, and water supply, which can change the nutrient profiles of foods. In regions where food insecurity is already well-established, climate change may affect crops to such an extent that even greater food insecurity follows.

Cons:

* The diet can be expensive.
* It is very high in saturated fat.
* It is low in fiber.
* It can be monotonous, which may make it difficult to follow in the long term.
* The current iteration of the diet recommends use of processed low-carb foods.
* It must be followed carefully in order for it to work.

Health rating: 6; Weight loss rating: 8

RAW FOOD DIET

Raw food diets have been around since the late 1800s when a doctor named Maximilian Bircher-Benner used a raw food diet as a treatment for patients in his sanatorium.

THE BASICS

People on raw food diets eat only whole foods that have not been heated above 115°F in order to preserve enzymes. It is mostly a plant-based diet. Foods included are fruits, vegetables, sea vegetables, nuts, seeds, and sprouts, as well as raw legumes and grains. While the majority of people following a raw food diet are vegan, some also eat raw animal proteins, raw eggs, and raw dairy products.

THE CLAIMS/BENEFITS

Raw foodists suggest that eating only raw foods has an alkalizing effect on the body. According to vegan raw food proponent Kimberly Snyder, when you eat an acidic diet of cooked foods, dairy products, and meats, it creates an acidic environment in your body. Because your body must return to its slightly alkaline state, when your body is acidic it draws minerals from your bones to return to alkalinity, thereby weakening the bones and increasing the risk of developing osteoporosis.

Raw foodists claim that disrupting the acid-alkaline balance in the body and bloodstream can cause an array of health problems, including weight gain and obesity, acid reflux, and buildup of toxins. The enzymes in raw foods also aid in digestion, which allows you to get the nutrients into your body quickly in order to improve health. According to raw foodists, a raw foods diet will confer the following benefits:

* Maintain the body's delicate acid-alkaline balance
* Promote a healthy weight
* Promote detoxification
* Reduce the risk of serious disease
* Improve digestion
* Maintain bone strength
* Improve overall health

NUTRITIONAL VALUE

A plant-based raw food diet is nutritionally dense. It is low in fat and tends to be low in calories. It is also moderately low in protein (unless you eat dairy products and animal proteins), and it is high in carbohydrates and fiber.

Choosing fruits and vegetables across the spectrum of colors and maintaining variety in your diet will help ensure you receive the vitamins and minerals you need. However, if you eat a vegan raw food diet, you may have difficulty getting vitamin B_{12}. Adding nutritional yeast or supplements will ensure you get this important vitamin.

SHORT-TERM EFFECTS

Short-term effects and risks of a raw food diet depend on the type of diet you choose. People consuming raw animal proteins, raw dairy, and raw eggs put themselves at risk of consuming dangerous foodborne bacteria such as *E. coli* and salmonella.

Raw vegan diets may induce weight loss in the short term due to calorie restriction. People on raw vegan diets may experience hunger, lack of satiation, gas, and bloating.

LONG-TERM EFFECTS

A raw food diet that is high in fruit and vegetable consumption may decrease the risk of developing a number of diseases, including certain cancers. Long-term use of a raw foods diet is associated with lowered cholesterol levels; however, this is true for both the "good" (HDL) and "bad" (LDL) cholesterol types. Long-term raw foodism also correlates with elevated levels of plasma homocysteine, which has been implicated in the development of atherosclerosis (plaque buildup in arteries) and vascular disease.

Those on raw food vegan diets may be deficient in vitamins B_{12} and D, as well as iron, zinc, selenium, and the omega-3 fatty acids DHA and EPA.

HEALTH AND WEIGHT LOSS RATING
The raw food diet has both benefits and drawbacks.

Pros:
* The plan contains plenty of fruits and vegetables.
* Weight loss is likely.
* No cooking time is required.

Cons:
* The diet's restrictive nature may make it difficult for some people to follow.
* The foods on the plan may require a great deal of prep time.
* Some foods may be unsafe eaten raw.
* The diet may lead to digestive problems.
* People may have difficulty finding adequate options when dining out.

Health rating: 5; Weight loss rating: 8

VEGAN/VEGETARIAN DIET

Vegans eat only plant-based foods, while vegetarians also include dairy products and eggs. None eat meat. Many cultures and people throughout history have pursued vegetarianism. Today, people on vegetarian diets typically cite one or more of three main reasons for pursuing a vegetarian diet: health, environment, and animal rights.

THE BASICS
Vegans do not consume or use any products derived from animals. This includes meat, dairy, eggs, fish and shellfish, poultry, honey, or any other animal-based foods. Like many omnivores, many vegans do enjoy processed foods. They often supplement protein in their diet by consuming soy-based products such as tofu.

Vegetarians may include eggs, dairy products, or both in their diet. Lacto-ovo vegetarians eat both eggs and dairy, while lacto vegetarians only eat dairy and ovo vegetarians only eat eggs. Vegans and vegetarians eat grains, legumes, fruits, vegetables, cereals, nuts, and seeds. They may also eat processed foods that do not contain animal products.

THE CLAIMS/BENEFITS

Proponents of a vegan or vegetarian diet claim a number of potential health benefits, including:

* Reduced risk of heart disease
* Reduced risk of developing certain cancers
* Weight control
* Reduced risk of developing chronic disease
* Improved energy

NUTRITIONAL VALUE

When a vegan diet consists primarily of whole foods, it is nutritionally dense. The diet tends to be low in calories and fat and high in fiber and carbohydrates. Vegans eating processed foods such as refined sugar or grains may be eating a less nutritious diet than those eating only whole foods. Protein in the vegan diet depends largely on the individual. Soy offers a complete protein to help boost protein levels. Vegan diets may also be low in vitamins B_{12} and vitamin D, as well as the omega-3 fatty acids EPA and DHA. Supplementation of these nutrients may be necessary. The diet is also low in cholesterol and saturated fat.

Vegetarian diets vary depending on what foods the vegetarian chooses. Lacto-ovo vegetarians may be eating quite a bit of saturated fat, especially if they incorporate cheese into their diet frequently. The diet tends to be high in carbohydrates and moderate in protein. Diets featuring heavy consumption of fruits and vegetables also tend to be nutritionally dense.

SHORT-TERM EFFECTS

The short-term effects of a vegan and vegetarian diet may have long-lasting health effects, according to a study evaluating the effects of a 10-day residential program in which 1,615 participants were fed only vegan foods. The study showed that in just 10 days on the program, participants

PRESERVING NUTRIENTS IN VEGETABLES WHEN COOKING

Vegetables can lose nutrients when they are cooked too long, at too high heat, or in the wrong manner. To preserve nutrients in vegetables when you cook them, choose a method such as steaming or microwaving. Steaming vegetables keeps the nutrients in the vegetables, while boiling them allows the nutrients to leach into the water, which you then discard. When microwaving, put the vegetables in a container with a small amount of water and cover them with plastic wrap. Roasting and grilling also preserve nutrients.

lost weight, lowered their blood pressure, lowered their blood sugar, and improved their blood lipid profiles.

People switching to a vegan or vegetarian diet from the Standard American Diet may initially experience gas or bloating as the body gets used to eating higher-fiber foods.

LONG-TERM EFFECTS

Vegans may not consume enough protein if they don't eat soy or take care to properly combine amino acids in foods. Vegans may be deficient in essential nutrients such as vitamins B_{12} and D. Vegan mothers who are deficient in B_{12} and breastfeed their babies may leave their children deficient in this vitamin as well, putting them at risk of failure to thrive and lack of proper brain development.

HEALTH AND WEIGHT LOSS RATING

With vegan and vegetarian diets, how healthy the diet is and whether you can lose weight on it depend largely upon the diet's implementation. They have many benefits and drawbacks.

Pros:
* These diets are low in saturated fat and cholesterol.
* They are high in healthy whole foods like fruits and vegetables.
* They are high in fiber.

Cons:
* You may feel hungry on these diets.
* These diets are restrictive and may be difficult to follow.
* Just because a food is vegan or vegetarian doesn't mean it is healthy. Many processed foods advertised as being vegan or vegetarian are high in sugar, sodium, additives, and preservatives.

Vegan *Health rating: 7; Weight loss rating: 6*
Vegetarian *Health rating: 5; Weight loss rating: 2*

KETOGENIC DIET

The ketogenic diet is a low-carbohydrate, high-fat diet designed to promote weight loss and better overall health. The diet is similar in macronutrient makeup to the Atkins diet, although its followers monitor the macronutrient ratios much more closely. It started as a diet to help people with epilepsy control seizures in the 1920s, but as medicines for the condition improved, fewer doctors recommend the diet any longer. While the ketogenic diet is still used by some doctors for epilepsy and other conditions, it has gained popularity recently as a weight loss diet.

THE BASICS

The ketogenic diet is high in fat, moderate in protein, and low in carbohydrates. Generally, the percentage of calories from each is 75 percent fat, 20 percent protein, and 5 percent carbohydrates. Carbohydrates come primarily from vegetables, and the diet eliminates or severely minimizes grains. No sugar is allowed. Protein comes from animal sources, while fat comes from added fats like olive oil, macadamia nut oil, avocado oil, coconut oil, and dairy fats, as well as from high-fat plant foods like avocados and nuts.

THE CLAIMS/BENEFITS

The ketogenic diet causes the body to burn stored body fat as fuel instead of burning glucose from carbohydrate intake. Burning fat in this manner produces ketones, which confer a number of benefits, including increased energy, decreased appetite, and fat loss. A ketogenic diet may also reduce seizures in people with epilepsy.

NUTRITIONAL VALUE

The ketogenic diet is high in fat, moderate in protein, and very low in carbohydrates. The foods are nutritionally dense, since the primary source of carbohydrates is vegetables. The diet is high in saturated fat and cholesterol. It is a sugar-free diet. The diet is low in fiber.

SHORT-TERM EFFECTS

A person switching from the Standard American Diet to a ketogenic diet may feel tired during the first week or so, as the body switches from burning glucose to running on ketones. These people may feel sluggish, or experience flu-like symptoms including aches and pains or headache.

SMALL MEALS

It used to be dietary wisdom that eating several small meals per day was more beneficial for weight loss than eating two or three larger ones. Recent studies show that there is no advantage to eating several small meals. Some people may find that eating more frequently, particularly when on a calorie-restricted diet, keeps them from getting hungry, while others do better with larger meals. If you suffer from acid reflux or GERD, then eating large meals increases abdominal pressure, which can cause flare-ups of heartburn. In that case, six small meals per day may be a better strategy.

Frequent urination is common during the first days, as is increased thirst. These effects pass within the first week. Rapid weight loss, primarily as a result of water loss, will occur within the first week of the diet. After that, weight loss will continue, but at a slower rate. People burning ketones may feel energized, and they may not have much of an appetite because ketones blunt the appetite.

LONG-TERM EFFECTS

Along with continued weight loss, more energy, and possible control of epileptic seizures, long-term followers of the ketogenic diet may experience constipation, and there is a slight risk of developing kidney stones. Although the diet is high in saturated fat and cholesterol, studies show that the diet improves blood lipid profiles by decreasing triglycerides and LDL and increasing HDL. It also decreases blood pressure. All of these correlate with a decreased risk of heart disease.

Because the ketogenic diet reduces blood sugar levels significantly, it may be helpful in preventing or controlling type 2 diabetes, although diabetics should monitor themselves for signs of ketoacidosis and work closely with their doctor.

HEALTH AND WEIGHT LOSS RATING

The ketogenic diet appears to have a lot going for it on both the health and weight loss fronts, but it may also have drawbacks.

Pros:
* The diet promotes weight loss, improved body composition, and decreased BMI.
* People find it highly satiating thanks to the fat in the diet.
* Ketones blunt hunger and increase energy.
* The diet has positive effects on heart disease risk factors.

Cons:
* The diet is restrictive and therefore may be difficult to follow.
* During the initial phases of the diet, flu-like symptoms may be demotivating.

Health rating: 6; Weight loss rating: 9

PALEO DIET

The paleo diet ostensibly has origins that extend all the way back to the earliest humans. The primary theory behind the paleo diet, as well as similar diets such as the Primal Blueprint, is that early humans were hunter-gatherers, so they ate only foods they could hunt and gather. Paleo experts theorize that modern humans have not evolved sufficiently to eat modern foods, and should instead stick to eating foods that are similar to what they would have hunted or gathered in order to obtain optimal health.

THE BASICS

People on paleo diets try to mimic the eating patterns of hunter-gatherers. To that end, they eat only whole, natural foods including fish, meat, poultry, nuts, seeds, vegetables, and fruits. They avoid processed foods, industrial seed oils like canola and grapeseed oil, grains, and legumes. They may also eat natural sweeteners such as honey and maple syrup, as well as pressed vegetable oils such as extra-virgin olive oil and coconut oil. People on the paleo diet avoid dairy products, while people on the Primal Blueprint diet consume organic dairy from grass-fed cattle. In general, people on the paleo diet opt for organic foods, as well as for grass-fed or pastured beef, free-range poultry, and other animal proteins not produced via factory farms.

The paleo diet is not necessarily a low-carb diet, although because it is grain and sugar-free, it is a reduced-carbohydrate diet.

THE CLAIMS/BENEFITS

The paleo diet eliminates all artificial ingredients that may cause illness or inflammation. It has a much better balance of omega-3 to omega-6 fatty acids than the Standard American Diet, so it is an anti-inflammatory diet. One version of the paleo diet, the autoimmune protocol (AIP), also suggests that eating an anti-inflammatory diet may help reduce symptoms of autoimmune diseases such as Hashimoto's thyroiditis, lupus, and rheumatoid arthritis. While it is not necessarily a weight loss diet, the paleo diet can also result in weight loss and improve athletic performance.

NUTRITIONAL VALUE

The diet is a nutritious one. When properly followed, your primary food source is organic plant foods, including fruits, vegetables, nuts, and seeds.

diets

BIG PORTIONS

Whether you eat six small meals or three larger meals, portion control is essential. Eating portions that are too big can lead to caloric intake that exceeds calories burned. Many people don't realize how large their portions really are when compared to a serving. A serving of meat or fish is 3 ounces, but many people believe a serving to be 6 ounces or more. Even if you eat larger portions in fewer meals, you still need to learn to control portions in order to maintain a healthy weight.

The diet contains moderate amounts of fiber and protein. Depending on how it is implemented, it can either be low or high in fat. The diet includes a balance of saturated, monounsaturated, and polyunsaturated fats, but it doesn't include trans fats. The diet allows no artificial ingredients. You can customize it to be low-carb and high-fat or high-carb and low-fat, based on your own individual needs and preferences.

SHORT-TERM EFFECTS

As you clean up your food intake and eliminate starchy grains, sugar, and processed foods, you may notice initial weight loss. One study showed that people following the paleo diet for 12 weeks improved their glucose tolerance. Other short-term studies showed decreased weight and BMI, decreased blood pressure, decreased triglycerides, and increased HDL.

LONG-TERM EFFECTS

Studies show that long-term effects of the paleo diet include sustained weight loss (provided the diet is maintained), as well as improved blood lipid profiles, resting glucose, and blood pressure. Few studies have been conducted into the effects of the paleo diet on autoimmune disease, although anecdotal reports and early evidence are promising.

HEALTH AND WEIGHT LOSS RATING

The paleo diet may confer certain health benefits. While it is not necessarily a weight loss diet, it does promote some weight loss, and it can be customized to be low-carb to improve weight loss.

Pros:
* The diet is anti-inflammatory.
* It promotes eating natural, organic, minimally processed foods.
* It is satiating because portion size is not limited.

Cons:
* The food can be prohibitively expensive.
* The diet may be difficult to follow.
* It is a restrictive diet, which may be demotivating for some.

Health rating: 8; Weight loss rating: 3

MEDITERRANEAN DIET

The Mediterranean diet evolved from about 5,000 years of local, healthful eating on the island of Crete in the Mediterranean. Ancel Keys, who also developed and promoted the lipid hypothesis of heart disease, became interested in the diet when he conducted his Seven Countries Study. He observed that men living in Crete had lower rates of heart disease than others, as well as lower rates of cancer and greater longevity. Keys made a study of the eating and exercise habits of the men of Crete, even living among them. As a result, he made recommendations for Americans to adopt a lifestyle similar to theirs. This gave birth to the Mediterranean diet, in which people choose to eat in a pattern similar to those living in Crete.

THE BASICS

The diet is designed for both optimal health and pleasurable eating, which makes it a more sustainable eating pattern for many. Instead of getting rid of entire categories of food like so many diets do, the Mediterranean diet offers a blueprint for healthy eating that recommends eating mostly plant foods, using olive oil instead of butter, reducing salt and using herbs and spices for flavor instead, eating red meat very sparingly and instead enjoying fish and poultry, and drinking moderate amounts of red wine.

THE CLAIMS/BENEFITS

The Mediterranean diet is a heart-healthy diet, which studies have shown to reduce the risk factors for heart disease such as cholesterol, triglycerides, and blood sugar. Studies also show a reduced risk of developing cancer, Alzheimer's, and other diseases. Other benefits include increased longevity, reduced levels of high blood pressure, and reduced rates of obesity. While it is not specifically a weight loss diet, it is a way of eating that allows you to control your weight as long as you control portions and watch calories.

NUTRITIONAL VALUE

The Mediterranean diet is a healthy diet. It is low in saturated fat, cholesterol, and sodium. It is high in healthy fruits and vegetables and therefore nutritionally dense and high in fiber. It is also high in antioxidants. By eating a variety of fruits, vegetables, and grains, the diet will meet all of your micronutrient needs. The diet also helps balance essential fatty acid

FOOD PRESERVATION

When preserving foods, it is important to process them in such a way that you eliminate the potential for growth of foodborne pathogens. Can foods using a high-heat pressure canner, and make sure to use sterile jars and lids. Process the foods exactly according to the canning directions, and always include acidic ingredients to discourage bacterial growth. Before storing home-canned goods, check to ensure that the jars have a tight vacuum seal. If freezing foods, store them in a tightly sealed container and label them with the date you froze them. Rotate preserved foods on a first-in, first-out basis.

ratios, promoting intake of healthy omega-3 fatty acids, as well as beneficial mono- and polyunsaturated fats. The diet is high in fiber and, with portion control, is moderate in protein, calories, and fat.

SHORT- AND LONG-TERM EFFECTS

The short- and long-term effects of the Mediterranean diet are similar. Studies show that following the Mediterranean diet for a few weeks can reduce inflammation in the body, and this effect continues for as long as you sustain the diet. Antioxidants reduce oxidative stress. Numerous studies also report that the diet improves blood lipid profiles, decreases blood pressure, and, when eaten as a moderate- to low-calorie diet, can also reduce weight and BMI. With its heart-healthy effects and reduction in cancer rates, the diet also correlates with greater longevity, as well as with reduced rates of chronic disease.

HEALTH AND WEIGHT LOSS RATING

There's no doubt that the Mediterranean diet is a very healthy diet. It contains a healthy balance from all food groups, including meals based around plant foods.

Pros
* The diet is very healthy, because it is low in saturated fat and high in plant foods.
* The foods are delicious, making it an easy diet to maintain.
* The diet doesn't eliminate any food group, so you won't feel deprived.
* It promotes moderation.
* Moderate exercise is an essential component of the diet.

Cons
* The diet isn't necessarily a weight loss diet.
* Portion control is necessary for weight loss and maintenance.

Health rating: 10; Weight loss rating: 5

WEIGHT WATCHERS

Weight Watchers is a commercial weight loss program that started in the 1970s. The program focuses on finding healthy ways to reduce calories and control portions in order to lose weight. It has always focused on providing a low-cost way for people to accomplish this.

THE BASICS

At its heart, the Weight Watchers program is a low-calorie diet. People on Weight Watchers lose weight via portion control and exercise. The program also provides support for members with weekly weigh-ins, as well as instructions on how to make lifestyle changes.

One of the reasons Weight Watchers has been so successful is that it doesn't restrict any foods or food groups. Instead, the program seeks to provide lower-calorie, portion-controlled offerings for favorite foods. People who subscribe to Weight Watchers can find these recipes on the Internet, in Weight Watchers cookbooks, and in the Weight Watchers magazine. The organization also produces a variety of premade portion-controlled, reduced-calorie foods, available at supermarkets.

Weight Watchers makes it easy for people to follow the program and remain within their food allowances for the day. Currently, it uses the Points and PointsPlus Programs, in which you have an allotted number of food points per day. When you have eaten all of your points, you are done eating for the day. Personalized coaching and group meetings help you understand the program and how it works.

THE CLAIMS/BENEFITS

Weight Watchers is exactly as advertised: it's about losing weight and maintaining that loss through portion control and reduced calories. Benefits of weight loss include increased energy, improved BMI and body composition, and possibly decreased risk of heart disease and certain cancers.

NUTRITIONAL VALUE

Weight Watchers has balanced offerings across all food groups. The diet is low in calories and contains adequate levels of micronutrients, although if you are primarily eating processed foods, supplementation may be necessary. Weight Watchers foods are low in fat, and thus tend to be lower in saturated fats and cholesterol than the Standard American Diet. Commercial offerings, which you don't have to make part of your program, may be high in sodium, and they may contain sugar, additives, preservatives, and artificial ingredients.

SHORT- AND LONG-TERM EFFECTS

A recent study showed that Weight Watchers was the most effective commercial weight loss plan, conferring modest weight loss to participants. Maintenance of results requires ongoing calorie restriction, portion control, and moderate activity levels.

Low-calorie diets work for most people, although for some they are not as effective as other types of diets. Studies show that low-calorie diets high in carbohydrates and sugar, such as the Weight Watchers diet, may increase LDL and total cholesterol, as well as triglycerides. Low-calorie diets pursued over the long term may also slow metabolism.

HEALTH AND WEIGHT LOSS RATING

Weight Watchers is a good all-in-one program that teaches you to make lifestyle changes for weight control. Of the commercial weight loss programs, studies indicate it is one of the most effective. The program, however, does have both benefits and drawbacks.

Pros:
* The program is easy to follow.
* It is easy to personalize.
* It allows a wide variety of foods.
* You can get as much support as you need.
* The program is affordable.

Cons:
* Low-calorie diets can leave you hungry.
* Foods and recipes contain sugar and salt.
* Any potential cardio-protective benefits most likely arise from loss of weight, and not from the healthfulness of the food.
* The diet allows for processed foods, and it's easy to make the diet consist entirely of processed foods.

Health rating: 4; Weight loss rating: 7

DASH

DASH is an acronym for Dietary Approaches to Stop Hypertension. Originally designed as a blood pressure–lowering diet, doctors now recommend it for heart health as well as weight loss. DASH is not a temporary diet, but rather a lifestyle intervention to reduce the risk of heart attack and stroke.

The National Heart, Lung, and Blood Institute at the National Institutes of Health developed the DASH diet as a flexible eating plan for people with high blood pressure.

THE BASICS

There are two levels of the DASH eating plan: the standard DASH diet and the lower-sodium DASH diet. Both call for significant lowering of sodium in the diet. The standard plan, which is for people without high blood pressure who wish to be healthier, aims to lower sodium intake to 2,300 mg or less per day. For people with high blood pressure, diabetes, or chronic kidney disease, or for African Americans and people over the age of 51, the lower-sodium DASH diet allows for 1,500 mg or less of sodium per day.

Other DASH guidelines include:

* Make fruits, vegetables, and fat-free or low-fat dairy the majority of your diet.
* Eat whole grains, seafood, poultry, beans, nuts, and seeds in moderation.
* Restrict sodium to less than 2,300 or 1,500 mg per day.
* Limit red meat, processed foods, processed grains, and sugar.
* Eat a variety of fruits and vegetables to get the macronutrients you need.

THE CLAIMS/BENEFITS

The DASH plan is designed to lower blood pressure, reduce the incidence of osteoporosis, lower the risk of heart disease and stroke, and prevent cancer and type 2 diabetes. Because it is a low-fat, low-calorie plan, it can also promote weight loss or help maintain a healthy weight.

NUTRITIONAL VALUE

The DASH diet has been designed in accordance with the scientifically created Dietary Guidelines for Americans, which are issued by the USDA and the Department of Health and Human Services. The DASH diet is a very healthy plan: low in saturated and trans fats, sodium, and sugar, and high in essential vitamins and minerals. It contains moderate levels of protein and fat and minimal processed foods, and is low in cholesterol.

SHORT- AND LONG-TERM EFFECTS

Studies show that the DASH diet is effective at lowering and controlling hypertension (high blood pressure). The diet is low in saturated fat, cholesterol, and sugar, which may also lower and keep blood lipid profiles within a healthy range, reducing the risk of cardiovascular disease and stroke. The nutrient-dense foods provide protection against a number of diseases. Because the diet emphasizes low-fat dairy products, it is rich in calcium and magnesium, which provide protective benefits to bones and may prevent osteoporosis.

HEALTH AND WEIGHT LOSS RATING

The DASH diet is designed based upon the best scientific evidence available. It follows the 2010 Nutritional Guidelines for Americans, which is the diet recommended by the National Institutes of Health. It is proven to be protective against developing hypertension, as well as lowering it in people who already have high blood pressure. While not necessarily a low-calorie diet, it can be customized for weight loss.

Pros:
* The diet is scientifically verified.
* It is effective at controlling hypertension.
* It reduces the risk of heart disease, stroke, and other diseases.
* It is easy to follow.
* The diet allows for a lot of variety.

Cons:

* The DASH diet is not necessarily a weight loss diet, so you will need to adjust activity levels and caloric intake to lose weight.
* Some studies show an increase in all-cause mortality with low-sodium diets. Talk to your doctor about the benefits or drawbacks of this type of a diet for your personal health situation.

Health rating: 10; Weight loss rating: 5

CHOOSING WISELY AT A RESTAURANT

The delicious menu items at restaurants may be tempting, but making nutritionally sound choices can help you maintain your health. If possible, read the restaurant menu ahead of time online so you know what to order when you visit the restaurant. Avoid deep-fried foods, as well as sugary drinks and desserts. Instead, choose lean proteins such as chicken or fish and order them alongside steamed vegetables. For a drink, have a glass of dry red wine, unsweetened iced tea, or water.

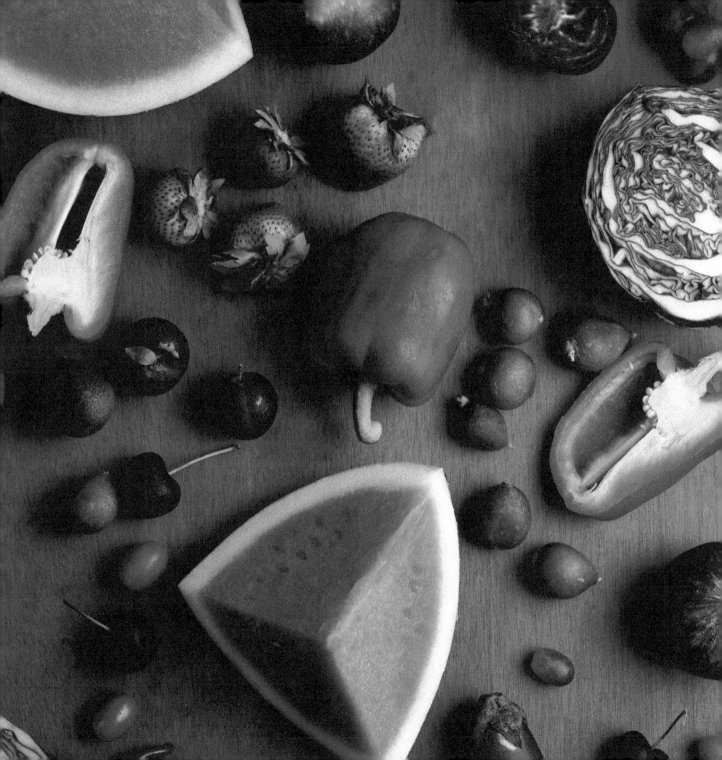

ailments
& allergies

The foods you eat affect the way you feel. Some foods do this by bolstering your body's natural immunity or providing the nutrients your body needs for optimal health. Others may soothe the body's inflammatory response. Still other foods may provide energy, aid in digestion, or prevent the buildup of excess stomach acid.

Certain foods may have a deleterious effect on your health. If you have sensitivities or allergies to certain foods, they may negatively affect your body by triggering inflammatory or immune system responses. Knowing your personal triggers for such responses is essential for maintaining proper health.

ailments

ailments

How various foods affect your health is uniquely individual. The effects of certain foods on your body have a lot to do with personal biology, genetics, and specific environmental factors. In general, however, eating whole, healthy foods such as fruits, vegetables, and lean meats will have an overall positive effect on your body. For common health complaints, employing nutritional strategies may offer relief from symptoms. It is also important that you work in close cooperation with your personal health care provider.

If you experience any of the following conditions, the suggested nutritional strategies may be helpful in conjunction with your regular health care.

ACID REFLUX (HEARTBURN, GERD)

Acid reflux, heartburn, and gastroesophageal reflux disease (GERD) occur when stomach acid passes through the lower esophageal sphincter and into the esophagus, causing a burning sensation and pain. Foods that trigger gastroesophageal reflux include those that increase pressure in the abdomen, those that weaken the lower esophageal sphincter, and those that increase stomach acid. With that in mind, engage the following nutritional strategies to improve symptoms of acid reflux:

* Avoid spicy foods, including avoiding onions, garlic, and chiles.
* Minimize fat by selecting lean meats, avoiding fried foods, and limiting added oils.
* Lower abdominal pressure by eating several small meals per day instead of three large meals.
* Avoid acidic foods, such as vinegar and citrus fruits.
* Avoid alcohol, coffee, and tea.
* For quick relief of indigestion or acid reflux, try swallowing a tablespoon of honey, sipping ginger tea or eating candied ginger, or chewing fennel seeds or fresh fennel.

ACNE

Excess oil production, clogged pores, and bacteria are the primary causes of acne, which occurs when a clogged pore forms an environment conducive to bacterial growth. The body's immune system responds with inflammation that erupts on the skin as acne.

Conventional wisdom used to suggest that eating fatty foods and chocolate caused or aggravated acne, but scientific studies do not support that hypothesis. While research is still ongoing, some evidence exists suggesting that highly processed grains and simple sugars may contribute to acne flare-ups.

Since acne is an inflammatory condition, an anti-inflammatory diet may help minimize flare-ups. Avoid inflammatory foods such as trans fats, refined carbohydrates, sugar, alcohol, artificial colors and flavors, preservatives, and foods high in omega-6 fatty acids. Instead, combat acne with an anti-inflammatory, whole-foods diet that contains plenty of fresh fruits and vegetables, along with lean proteins such as fish and poultry, low-glycemic grains, walnuts, and omega-3 fatty acids.

AMENORRHEA (ABSENT PERIODS)

Amenorrhea is the condition that occurs when women of menstruating age do not have periods. It is not the same as menopause (see page 189) and has distinctly different causes. There are two types of amenorrhea: primary and secondary. Primary amenorrhea occurs when a female reaches the age of 16 without onset of menstruation. Secondary amenorrhea occurs in a woman who used to have normal periods but misses three in a row.

A number of factors may cause primary and secondary amenorrhea, including anorexia, stress, hormone imbalances, too much exercise, and medications. Women experiencing amenorrhea should consult with their physician. Dietary approaches may help as well:

* If low body weight is the cause of amenorrhea, eat a diet that is adequate in calories to sustain or gain weight.
* Eat foods rich in vitamins D and K, calcium, and magnesium. Dairy products are an excellent source of these nutrients.

* Consume foods high in vitamin B_6, such as fish and leafy greens.
* Eat foods containing omega-3 fatty acids, such as seafood and flaxseed.
* Minimize processed foods, refined carbohydrates, and sugar.
* Avoid caffeine and alcohol.

ANEMIA

Anemia occurs when your blood doesn't contain enough healthy red cells to carry and deliver oxygen. Anemia has several causes, including blood loss and nutritional issues. Many nutrients are necessary to build blood cells, including iron, copper, vitamin E, and vitamins B_2, B_6, B_9, and B_{12}.

Consider the following nutritional strategies for anemia:

* You may need to supplement iron, as well as eat a diet that is rich in foods containing iron, such as clams, beef, organ meats, lamb, dark leafy greens, parsley, and kidney beans.
* Vitamin C enhances iron absorption. Eat vitamin C foods along with iron-containing foods, including citrus fruits, berries, kiwi, and dark leafy greens.
* Eat copper-rich foods such as dark leafy greens, legumes, and nuts.
* If you are a vegetarian and don't eat meat, you'll need to supplement B vitamins or eat foods fortified with B vitamins, such as soymilk or nutritional yeast.
* Eat foods high in vitamin E, such as nuts, seeds, and dark leafy greens.

ANXIETY

Anxiety takes many forms, such as social anxiety, phobias, generalized anxiety, among others. According to the Physician's Committee for Responsible Medicine, dietary considerations can influence mood, which may exacerbate the symptoms of anxiety disorders:

- Avoid caffeine, which is a central nervous system stimulant that can increase feelings of anxiety.
- Avoid alcohol, which is a central nervous system depressant and can increase feelings of sadness or depression.
- Keep blood sugar steady throughout the day by eating breakfast and regular meals. Include protein at every meal.
- Eat complex carbohydrates, such as whole grains, which release the neurotransmitter serotonin to calm anxiety. Try foods such as quinoa, brown rice, and oatmeal.
- Drink plenty of water, since hydration has an effect on mood.
- Eat a balanced diet that minimizes sugar, processed foods, and refined carbohydrates such as white flour.

ARTHRITIS

Arthritis is an inflammatory condition that causes pain and swelling in the joints. Along with medical treatment, eating a diet rich in anti-inflammatory foods and avoiding foods that may cause inflammation can help ease the pain and symptoms of arthritis.

- Eat a Mediterranean-style diet (see page 155), which may reduce inflammation.
- Avoid fried foods and meats cooked at high temperatures. These foods have been shown to contribute to inflammation because they generate something called advanced glycation end products (AGEs). High levels of AGEs may trigger inflammation.
- Avoid sugar, refined carbohydrates, and processed foods.
- Eat whole, healthy foods such as fruits and vegetables, whole grains, nuts, seeds, and seafood.
- Try to eat between 27 and 28 grams of fiber per day to reduce inflammation. Studies show that eating this amount of fiber reduces the levels of C-reactive protein, which is a marker of inflammation.
- Drink alcohol, such as red wine, in moderation.

ATTENTION DEFICIT DISORDER (ADD) AND ATTENTION DEFICIT HYPERACTIVITY DISORDER (ADHD)

Both adults and children with ADD and ADHD may experience greatly relieved symptoms by following a dietary approach in conjunction with a medical approach prescribed by their doctors.

Some foods seem to correlate with ADD and ADHD symptoms, including those with artificial ingredients. Because of this correlation, it is best to choose whole, natural foods that are minimally processed. Avoid foods with chemical additives such as artificial flavors and colors, as well as those with preservatives. Provide fruits and vegetables, whole grains, dairy products, lean animal proteins, fish, nuts, and seeds as the cornerstones of a diet for someone with ADD or ADHD.

In some cases, vitamin and mineral deficiencies seem to correlate with ADD or ADHD. Choose foods high in zinc, such as pumpkin seeds and sesame seeds; foods high in iron, such as dark leafy greens and animal proteins; foods high in magnesium, such as yogurt, avocados, and black beans; and foods high in vitamin B_6, such as poultry, fish, and dark leafy greens.

AUTOIMMUNE DISEASES

Autoimmune diseases are a cluster of diseases in which the immune system attacks healthy cells in the body. There are over 80 types of autoimmune diseases, including lupus, rheumatoid arthritis, celiac disease, Hashimoto's thyroiditis, and many others.

Many doctors recommend that patients with autoimmune diseases eat an anti-inflammatory diet that is low in hydrogenated and trans fats, refined oils, processed carbs and sugar, red meat, and common allergens, but contains fresh fruits and vegetables, lean animal proteins, and healthy fats.

One dietary approach that seems to help people with autoimmune disease is the paleo autoimmune Protocol (AIP). The diet is a modified version of the paleo diet (see page 153), which eliminates all possible food triggers of inflammation and then allows you to gradually introduce them back into your diet to determine your own triggers. Along with traditional paleo guidelines, the AIP omits eggs, nuts, seeds, nightshades, alcohol, stevia, and thickeners such as guar gum from the diets. As your symptoms abate, you can begin to reintroduce these foods one at a time to determine your own personal triggers.

AUTISM/ASPERGER'S SYNDROME

Children and adults who fall on the autism spectrum may process casein and gluten differently than other people. Because of this, some people believe that feeding someone on the autism spectrum a diet that is free of gluten and casein may be helpful in alleviating some of the symptoms. While this theory has not yet been borne out by research, anecdotal evidence suggests that, at least in some cases, the diet may help to some extent.

Gluten is a sticky protein found in wheat, rye, and barley, while casein is a sticky protein found in dairy products. It can also be found in butter with additives and some types of margarine. Both gluten and casein find their way into a number of processed foods as well, so reading ingredients labels is essential.

Along with eliminating gluten and casein, choose a plant-based diet with moderate amounts of lean protein, healthy whole grains, plenty of fresh fruits and vegetables, and legumes. Avoid sugar, alcohol, caffeine, and artificial ingredients.

BACK PAIN

Back pain can occur for a number of reasons. For example, an autoimmune disease called ankylosing spondylitis may cause vertebral fusion, resulting in pain, or chronic stress might cause muscle spasms that in turn lead to pain.

Doctors, chiropractors, massage therapists, and physical therapists can all provide a program to help with back pain, but a nutritional approach may help as well:

* If your pain comes from an autoimmune disorder, then try an anti-inflammatory diet or the paleo (AIP, see page 169) to help lessen symptoms.
* Nutritional deficiencies can lead to muscular spasms, including back spasm. Increasing intake of calcium, magnesium, and

potassium may help balance electrolytes, which contract and relax muscles. Eat foods rich in these minerals such as low-fat dairy products, bananas, and dark leafy greens.

* Avoid caffeine and alcohol, which can exacerbate spasms and increase stress that causes you to tighten or clench muscles.

* To prevent back pain, eat a whole-foods diet that is nutrient-dense. Be sure to include vitamin D in fortified milk or get plenty of sunlight, since vitamin D helps the bones absorb calcium to keep them strong. Strong bones help build a healthy back. Other vitamins necessary for a healthy back include B_{12}, C, K, and E.

BRUISES

Bruises, or contusions, occur in your soft tissues. An injury causes blood vessels to break, and that blood can pool under the skin to form a dark bruise. If you've had a visible injury, then some bruising is understandable. However, if you bruise easily without injury, then there might be other causes at play, such as blood-thinning medications, which will likely make you bruise more easily. If you aren't taking such medications, bruising easily may be a result of nutritional deficiencies.

One nutritional cause of bruising is vitamin C deficiency. To combat it, eat foods high in vitamin C, such as citrus fruits, berries, and dark leafy greens. A vitamin K deficiency might also be the culprit. Vitamin K is a vitamin that is responsible for blood clotting; in the absence of vitamin K, blood does not clot. You can get vitamin K in dark leafy greens and cruciferous vegetables, as well as from animal sources such as organ meats.

CANCER

If you have been diagnosed with any form of cancer, it is essential to work with your health care providers to receive the best possible treatment. You can also use nutritional solutions to supplement your recovery, helping you stay strong while you undergo treatment.

The American Cancer Society recommends eating a plant-based nutrient-dense diet of whole foods to help maintain your strength. Include at least 2½ cups of fresh fruits and vegetables daily, selecting foods in a variety of colors to meet your nutrient needs. These foods not only contain vitamins and minerals, but they contain phytonutrients and antioxidants that fight disease and inflammation. The American Cancer Society also recommends limiting unhealthy foods in your diet, such as deep-fried foods, processed foods, sugar, trans fats, and fatty animal proteins.

Although you may feel nauseated from your cancer treatment, try to avoid skipping meals, as your body needs nutrition. Avoid substances that may interact with treatment medications, such as caffeine and alcohol.

CELIAC DISEASE

Celiac disease is an autoimmune condition in which the body perceives gluten as a foreign invader and begins to attack the intestinal villi. This causes damage to the small intestine and makes it difficult to absorb nutrients from foods. For people with celiac disease, even trace amounts of gluten can cause intestinal damage, so it is important to completely avoid it. Gluten is a sticky protein found in wheat, barley, and rye. It is also present in many other foods, including soy sauce, many types of mustard, and a number of other foods. People with celiac disease need to take care to avoid cross-contamination when preparing foods or eating in restaurants.

While there is no cure for celiac disease, completely removing gluten from the diet does control it. Because damage to intestinal villi occurs each time one consumes gluten, nutrient absorption is often an issue. As you eliminate gluten from your diet, you should eat high-quality, nutrient-dense whole foods in order to renourish your body. Since this is an autoimmune condition, some people with celiac disease successfully follow the paleo (AIP, see page 153), which may help with intestinal healing.

COLD SORES

Cold sores, also known as fever blisters, commonly occur on or around the lips, as well as inside the mouth or gums. The herpes simplex virus type 1 (HSV-1) causes cold sores. The virus can remain dormant for years, only to flare up again. While little research exists supporting nutritional approaches to either HSV-1 or the herpes simplex virus type 2 (HSV-2), which causes genital herpes, there is a body of anecdotal evidence suggesting that eating foods high in the amino acid arginine may trigger outbreaks. Foods containing high amounts of arginine include chocolate, nuts, and oats.

To counteract arginine in foods, Dr. Andrew Weil recommends eating foods that are high in the amino acid lysine. These foods include fruits and vegetables, dairy products, eggs, brewer's yeast, sprouts, and fish.

Along with limiting arginine or balancing it with lysine-containing foods, you should also eat a diet rich in antioxidants to keep your immune system working to fight cold sore outbreaks.

COLDS

There's all sorts of conventional nutritional wisdom available for fighting the common cold, such as "feed the cold and starve the fever," take lots of vitamin C, and eat chicken soup.

When you have a cold, you stand the best chance of recovering quickly when you provide your body with the nutrition it needs for good health. To prevent colds, and to possibly help shorten their duration, eat foods that are high in antioxidant vitamins, such as vitamins C and E and beta-carotene. Include plenty of fresh fruits and vegetables, but avoid drinking too much juice, which is high in sugar. Foods that have plenty of antioxidants include citrus fruits, cherries, and cruciferous vegetables, among many others.

Staying hydrated is important, so drink plenty of water. You should also eat foods containing zinc, such as eggs and whole grains. There is some truth to eating chicken soup if you have a cold. The soup helps thin mucus and lessen congestion, and its warmth may be soothing to a sore throat.

CONSTIPATION

According to the National Institutes of Health, if you have fewer than three bowel movements in a week, then you are constipated. Constipation may have a number of causes, such as inadequate fiber in the diet, dehydration, certain medications, and stress. Fortunately, most cases of constipation are easy to clear up with dietary strategies.

An age-old home remedy for constipation is drinking prune juice, which often works well. Prunes and prune juice act naturally as a laxative to get things moving. Eating foods high in magnesium or supplementing magnesium can also help, because magnesium serves to relax intestinal walls, allowing stool to move through them. Foods high in magnesium include dark leafy greens, pumpkin seeds, and yogurt.

If you're constipated, avoiding eating dairy foods and heavy animal proteins. Instead, drink plenty of water and eat foods high in fiber, including legumes, whole grains, fruits, and vegetables.

COUGH

A persistent cough can be very irritating. Whether you are coughing as a result of a common cold or allergies, or you have a more serious condition such as bronchitis, what you eat can either soothe or irritate your cough.

Coughs typically occur either as the result of irritation in the throat, or because of mucus in the chest. Eating hot, comforting foods such as soup or drinking hot tea can thin the mucus, making it easier to cough up. Spicy foods, such as hot chiles or black pepper, may also thin mucus, as can drinking plenty of fluids. To soothe an irritated cough, try a tablespoon of organic raw honey, or mix honey and lemon juice into a cup of warm water for a soothing alcohol-free hot toddy. Adding a little thyme may serve as an expectorant.

Finally, build up your immune system by eating nutrient-dense foods that are high in antioxidant vitamins, such as vitamins C and E and beta-carotene.

DANDRUFF

Dandruff may be itchy and irritating, but it isn't life-threatening. Still, nobody wants an itchy scalp, and most people can do without those white flakes. While the exact causes of dandruff remain unknown, many things are thought to contribute to the condition, including oily skin, hormones, and yeast. Nutrient deficiencies may also contribute to the problem.

Along with using a shampoo formulated to control dandruff, you may want to consider a nutritional approach. Dandruff may be the result of nutrient deficiencies, including nutrients such as zinc, essential fatty acids, vitamin C, or vitamin B_6. Just as these deficiencies can show up on your skin, they can also appear on your scalp as hair loss, dandruff, or other issues. To ensure a healthy scalp, eat nutrient-rich foods that contain vitamin C, such as leafy greens and citrus fruits. Foods high in vitamin B_6 include fish, poultry, and legumes. For essential fatty acids, eat nuts, seeds, whole grains, and seafood. Drink plenty of water as well, to keep the scalp healthy and hydrated, and avoid sugar, which can feed yeast and allow it to proliferate.

DEPRESSION

Research shows that depression has a biochemical basis as well as an emotional one. Because the foods you eat have a profound effect on your body and your brain's biochemistry, how you eat can affect depression.

B vitamins are necessary for the production of mood chemicals in the brain, and deficiencies of these vitamins may increase symptoms of depression. Of the B vitamins, folate and B_{12} have the largest role to play, so it is important that your diet contains adequate levels of folate, vitamin B_{12}, and other B-complex vitamins. You can get these vitamins from animal protein as well as from fortified foods and nutritional yeast.

Research also indicates that omega-3 fatty acids may help reduce symptoms of depression. You can get omega-3 fatty acids in fish and seafood, as well as from vegetable sources like walnuts and chia seeds. You can also supplement with fish oil or other forms of omega-3 fatty acids. Talk to your doctor about how supplementation may interact with any of your medications.

DIABETES, TYPE 2

Type 2 diabetes occurs, typically in adults, when the body no longer uses insulin properly, preventing the body from keeping blood glucose levels under control. People diagnosed with diabetes may require medication to help control blood sugar, or they may be able to control symptoms strictly through diet.

Different nutritional approaches may be helpful for managing symptoms. It is important to work with your physician to find the approach that works for you.

One form of diabetes diet is a low-carbohydrate diet, which studies have shown to be just as effective at managing diabetes symptoms as low-fat and low-glycemic diets. People selecting this form of diabetes management should avoid foods high in carbohydrates such as grains, sugar, and legumes, focusing instead on proteins, vegetables, and fats to make up the bulk of their diet.

Another approach is to eat a calorie-controlled diet that manages blood sugar via complex carbohydrates, fruits and vegetables, low-fat dairy, and lean protein.

DIARRHEA

Diarrhea carries with it the risk of dehydration, especially in children or elderly people. It is usually associated with acute stomach issues such as gastroenteritis or food poisoning, or with chronic conditions such as irritable bowel syndrome (see page 185) or celiac disease (see page 171).

For acute diarrhea arising from gastroenteritis or food poisoning, the BRAT diet is one of the best solutions. The BRAT diet contains only bland foods that soothe the stomach. During the time that you are experiencing diarrhea, eat only bananas, rice, applesauce, and toast (BRAT). These foods will help solidify the stool, and they contain potassium to replace lost electrolytes. Drink plenty of water as well, to rehydrate yourself.

Avoid fried or greasy foods, as well as fruits and vegetables that may irritate a sensitive stomach or cause gas. These include peppers, onions, broccoli, garlic, and other "roughage" vegetables. You should also skip caffeine and alcohol, both of which may irritate your stomach.

DYSMENORRHEA (PAINFUL PERIODS)

Severe menstrual pain is not only uncomfortable, but it can severely decrease quality of life during the days you have your period. While hot water bottles and NSAIDs can help, nutritional approaches may also help soothe menstrual pain. For best results, you should pursue these strategies throughout the month, even when you don't have your period:

* Eliminate caffeine, which can contribute to breast tenderness and uterine cramping.
* The hormone estrogen is partially responsible for cramping. To lower estrogen levels, eat foods lower in fat.
* Focus on a plant-based diet, avoiding animal products. If you do eat meat, dairy products, or eggs, choose those that have been raised without hormones to help keep hormones at natural levels.
* Eating plenty of fiber also reduces estrogen levels. Try high-fiber foods such as legumes, whole grains, fruits, and vegetables.

EAR INFECTION

Many children experience chronic ear infections. While there are a number of medical treatments for ear infections that include surgical placement of tubes and the use of antibiotics, seeking a nutritional approach may help reduce the duration or incidence of ear infections.

Ear infections are caused by bacteria that are trapped in the ear canal. When a doctor treats the bacterial infection with antibiotics, those medications kill both harmful and beneficial bacteria. Therefore, it is important to replace the beneficial bacteria after a bout of antibiotics. Adding fermented foods such as yogurt or kefir to your diet can replace these beneficial bacteria. Flavor these foods with natural fruits that don't include sugar, as sugar can feed the growth of harmful bacteria.

Choose foods that build the immune system. Those foods include fresh fruits and vegetables that are high in micronutrients, as well as healthy whole grains, legumes, nuts, seeds, low-fat dairy products, and lean animal proteins.

ECZEMA

Eczema is an inflammatory condition that affects the skin. The condition is chronic and recurring. Outbreaks of eczema can be uncomfortable and painful, as well as embarrassing.

Eczema flare-ups may occur as a result of ingesting foods to which you are allergic (see common allergens, starting on page 195). Work with your doctor on an elimination diet to discover your own food triggers and avoid those foods assiduously. Some foods associated with triggering eczema include tomatoes, soy, dairy products, wheat, and peanuts.

Eating a diet high in vitamin C, omega-3 fatty acids, and flavonoids (found in dark berries) may also help calm eczema. Supplementing probiotics or eating fermented foods may help too.

FATIGUE

Fatigue can have numerous causes, including lack of sleep, stress, illness, anemia (see page 166), and improper diet or malnutrition. Taking care of fatigue includes treating the underlying cause of the issue. However, there are also nutritional approaches you can take.

Many people's first response to fatigue is to ingest some caffeine in the form of coffee, tea, or an energy drink. Using caffeine regularly may give you an initial jolt of energy, but it may wear off quickly, or you may require more caffeine for the same effects as you develop a tolerance to it. Caffeine can increase fatigue, especially when you first begin to go through withdrawal. Quitting caffeine may be difficult at first, but in the long run you will notice increased energy levels.

Eating sugar and refined carbohydrates can also cause fatigue because sugar gives you a quick rush as blood glucose levels rise, followed by a crash when they fall. Avoiding these rises and falls of blood sugar can help you feel alert throughout the day.

The best way to control fatigue is eating a diet consisting of healthy, unprocessed foods and getting plenty of sleep.

FEVER

Should you really starve a fever, as the old adage suggests? When your body spikes a fever, it is doing so as an immune response to fight off a bacterial infection or a virus. As your fever rises, so does your body temperature, which increases your body's energetic needs. If you can bring yourself to do so, you might try to give yourself some energy in the form of food or drink to meet your body's needs. Choose easy-to-swallow yet nutritious foods such as 100 percent pure juice or broth. Herbal teas may also be soothing. If your stomach is upset as well, or if you have diarrhea, stick to the BRAT diet (see page 175) to soothe your stomach. Avoid caffeine and alcohol, but drink plenty of fluids, especially water, to replenish liquids lost via sweating.

FIBROMYALGIA

People with fibromyalgia experience chronic pain and overwhelming fatigue. These symptoms resemble many of those associated with autoimmune diseases such as rheumatoid arthritis, celiac disease, and lupus. With this similarity in symptoms, some people with fibromyalgia follow the paleo (AIP, see page 153), which eliminates all processed foods, legumes, grains, industrial seed oils, dairy, and nightshades, and focuses on whole, organic fruits and vegetables, as well as grass-fed, pastured, and wild-caught organic meat and seafood, nuts, and seeds.

If unable to follow a strict AIP, people with fibromyalgia may still want to avoid certain foods that seem to exacerbate symptoms, including artificial sweeteners like aspartame (NutraSweet) and sucralose (Splenda). Other foods to consider avoiding include artificial colors and flavors, MSG, simple carbs and sugars, nightshades, gluten, dairy, and caffeine. Eliminating these foods from your diet may help minimize symptoms or prevent symptoms from worsening.

FOOD POISONING

Food poisoning is usually acute, coming on quickly within a few hours after eating the food containing the foodborne pathogen. It can occur with or without a fever, and symptoms resemble that of gastroenteritis, including diarrhea, vomiting, nausea, dizziness, sweating, abdominal pain, and weakness.

The last thing you may want to do when you have food poisoning is eat or drink, particularly if you are vomiting. However, vomiting and diarrhea can lead to dehydration and electrolyte imbalances, so as soon as you are able, you should try to at least drink clear fluids. Introduce fluids when you are able by first sucking on ice chips. If those stay down, you may proceed to drinking small amounts of water or apple juice, as well as bland foods such as soda crackers.

If diarrhea persists after vomiting ceases, follow the BRAT diet (see page 175) to allow your stomach time to heal. If symptoms continue for more than a day, consult your health care provider.

GALLSTONES/GALLBLADDER ATTACKS

Many people develop gallstones but remain asymptomatic. In some cases, gallstones can trigger painful gallbladder attacks that are extremely uncomfortable. While surgery is an option, you can also take dietary steps to minimize symptoms.

Diet may play a role in the formation of gallstones. To prevent them from forming, try to minimize dietary cholesterol, which can mix with bile salts to form stones. Minimize saturated fat intake and eat a diet that is high in fiber.

If you already have gallbladder issues or gallstones, certain foods can trigger attacks. To reduce symptoms, the University of Maryland Medical Center suggests avoiding very high-fat foods, including fried foods, full-fat dairy products, fatty cuts of meat, and processed foods. Eat a diet that is high in natural foods like fruits and vegetables and contains an adequate number of calories (between 1,800 and 2,200 depending on your age, sex, weight, and activity levels).

GAS

If you tend to be someone who burps or passes gas a lot, then you might want to consider a diet that helps minimize gassiness. Gassiness occurs for a number of reasons, including swallowing air, fermentation of bacteria in the belly, and eating foods that are difficult to digest. As gas builds up, you need to release it or it will cause bloating, pain, and cramps.

Certain foods are notoriously gassy foods. These include carbonated beverages, which contribute their own gas to the digestive tract, and fatty foods that delay stomach emptying. Foods that empty slowly from the stomach and tend to ferment also include legumes, cruciferous vegetables, grains, and foods that contain sugar alcohols like mannitol, sorbitol, and xylitol. Dairy products may also cause gas if you are lactose-intolerant.

To minimize gas, soak and rinse legumes before cooking them. Eat gassy foods slowly and in moderation, and minimize fatty and fried foods. If you have lactose intolerance, avoid dairy products or use lactose-free milk.

GASTROENTERITIS (STOMACH FLU)

Gastroenteritis can hit quickly, and it can be quite severe. Characterized by fever, vomiting, and diarrhea, gastroenteritis doesn't often stay long, but it can leave you weak, shaky, and just feeling awful.

During the acute phase of gastroenteritis, all you can really do is ride it out. Don't try to introduce food or liquid until vomiting has passed. Be careful to avoid dehydration. If you remain unable to keep liquids down for more than 24 hours, seek medical care. Once vomiting has ceased, start introducing liquids by sucking on ice chips and taking sips of water. Once you are certain that it will stay down, try a little bit of apple juice and something very bland such as soda crackers. When you do return to eating, start with very mild foods such as dry toast or chicken broth, because your stomach is likely to be tender. If you have diarrhea, follow the BRAT diet (see page 175).

GOUT

Gout is a painful condition that results from uric acid in the bloodstream forming painful crystals. These crystals accumulate around joints, causing pain that is often severe. Foods high in a substance called purine can cause the buildup of uric acid in the blood. While you can eat these foods in moderation, you should eat them in conjunction with foods that help to minimize their effects. These additional tips will help:

* Avoid organ meats.
* Eat plenty of healthy fruits and vegetables. Even high-purine vegetables don't seem to affect blood levels of uric acid significantly.
* Avoid seafood high in purines, such as scallops, trout, sardines, tuna, herring, mackerel, and anchovies. Other seafood is fine.
* Eat foods high in vitamin C, which may lower levels of uric acid. Include dark leafy greens, berries, and citrus fruits.
* Don't drink alcohol, because it can increase uric acid levels.
* Moderate, but don't avoid, foods that contain moderate levels of purines, such as legumes.
* Drink plenty of water to keep hydrated and dilute uric acid levels in the blood.

HAIR LOSS

Hair loss may occur for a number of reasons. It may be the result of hypothyroidism, hyperthyroidism, hormonal changes, stress, or as a side effect of medications you may be taking. Some hair loss is not preventable. However, eating nourishing foods can help keep the follicles in your scalp healthy, which may prevent or slow down hair loss from preventable causes.

Including fish and shellfish in your diet may help you maintain a healthy scalp. Fish is one of the best sources of omega-3 fatty acids, which improve the condition of the scalp, and it is also a major source of vitamin B_5, also known as pantothenic acid. While more research is required, there is some evidence that pantothenic acid can help prevent hair thinning and loss. Try to include fish in your diet at least three times per week.

HALITOSIS

Halitosis, or bad breath, can be socially embarrassing. It may have a number of causes, which may be related to the foods you eat, dehydration, poor dental hygiene, medication, and health issues such as diabetes.

While proper dental hygiene is the first step in managing bad breath, dietary solutions may help, too. To avoid temporary bad breath, skip foods with strong odors such as onions and garlic, which can linger for hours, or even a few days after eating them, in spite of brushing your teeth.

For consistent bad breath, other dietary interventions may be necessary. Drink plenty of water to remain hydrated, and eat foods high in antioxidants to neutralize bacteria that may be contributing to bad breath. You should also eat foods that neutralize bad breath, including yogurt, fibrous and crunchy fruits and vegetables like apples and celery, fresh herbs that are rich in chlorophyll like parsley and mint, ginger, fruits with enzymes such as papaya, and fennel seeds. Because chronic bad breath may be linked to other health issues, you may also want to consult your health care provider.

HEADACHES

Headaches, particularly migraines, may have a multitude of food triggers. Because these foods don't trigger headaches every time, and because the triggers vary greatly from person to person, scientific evidence is difficult to establish. However, many people have noted anecdotally that some common foods seem to correlate with the onset of migraine headaches, including caffeine, alcohol, and chocolate. If these are food triggers for you, it is best to avoid them.

Two other groups of foods seem to be migraine triggers as well. These include foods that contain tannins, such as red wine, beer, tea, and smoked foods. Foods with tyramine may also be triggers. These include avocados, aged cheeses, and cured meats.

The National Headache Foundation recommends following a diet low in processed foods, sugars, and artificial ingredients, minimizing alcohol and caffeine intake, and drinking plenty of water.

HYPERCHOLESTEROLEMIA (HIGH CHOLESTEROL)

High cholesterol is one of the risk factors for heart disease. Cholesterol is a waxy substance made in the liver, and your body uses it for many important functions. Cholesterol provides structure to cells, and it is necessary for brain function and hormone production. Your body produces two types of cholesterol, HDL (the so-called "good" cholesterol), and LDL ("bad" cholesterol). Doctors strive to have people increase HDL levels while lowering LDL and total cholesterol. Diet can have an influence on this.

If you have been diagnosed with high cholesterol, the following nutritional interventions may help:

* Eat foods that contain soluble fiber, such as oats, oat bran, legumes, and other whole grains. Soluble fiber has been shown to lower both LDL and total cholesterol numbers.
* Eat plenty of plant foods. Plants contain sterols and stanols, substances that block dietary cholesterol absorption.
* Eat foods rich in omega-3 fatty acids, such as fish and walnuts. Omega-3 fats have been shown to boost HDL cholesterol.
* Avoid foods that contain trans fats.
* Replace saturated animal fats with unsaturated vegetable fats such as extra-virgin olive oil and avocado oil.

HYPERTENSION (HIGH BLOOD PRESSURE)

Uncontrolled high blood pressure increases the risk of stroke and heart disease because it weakens blood vessels. The DASH diet (see page 159) is low in fat and sodium and high in plant foods, and it has been shown to bring about a quick reduction in blood pressure.

Some foods may increase blood pressure, including alcohol, salt, refined carbohydrates and sugar, and caffeine. Avoiding these foods may help lower your blood pressure. Eating high-fiber, nutrient-dense plant foods may also help. Eat a diet rich in plant foods such as whole grains, legumes, nuts and seeds, fruits, vegetables, fish, and poultry. Since losing weight can also help lower blood pressure, if you are overweight, try a calorie-controlled diet to reduce your weight.

A diet low in calcium, vitamin D, and magnesium may also raise blood pressure, so it is important to eat foods that contain these vitamins. Low-fat dairy products contain these vitamins, so consuming them may help reduce hypertension.

HYPOTENSION (LOW BLOOD PRESSURE)

Low blood pressure may cause dizziness, especially with positional changes. A reading of 90/60 is considered low blood pressure. For some people with a condition called postprandial hypotension, eating causes a drop in pressure. For postprandial hypotension, eat several small low-carb meals, and drink at least 12 ounces of water about 15 minutes before eating.

For people with generalized low blood pressure, don't eat a low-sodium diet. Try adding a bit of salt to your meals, or use salty ingredients such as soy sauce. Drink plenty of water, and eat a diet high in plant foods, dairy products, and lean animal proteins.

HYPERTHYROIDISM (OVERACTIVE THYROID)

Hyperthyroidism occurs when the thyroid gland makes an excessive quantity of thyroid hormones. This can cause hormonal imbalances in the body that lead to a high metabolic state, and it may induce anxiety, rapid heartbeat, irritability, and sleeplessness, among other symptoms. The most common cause of hyperthyroidism is Graves' disease, which is an autoimmune condition.

For people who have autoimmune hyperthyroidism (Graves' disease), the paleo AIP (see page 153) may be helpful to reduce inflammation and improve the health of the gut. Goitrogens are foods that block the production of thyroid hormones, so for people who produce too much, these foods may be beneficial. Goitrogens include cruciferous vegetables like broccoli, mustard, and radishes, as well as soy.

Because hyperthyroidism can ultimately weaken bones, eating foods high in bone-building minerals such as calcium, magnesium, and vitamin D is also essential. Low-fat dairy products are an excellent source of these, as are dark leafy green vegetables.

HYPOTHYROIDISM (UNDERACTIVE THYROID)

When the thyroid gland doesn't create enough thyroid hormones, hypothyroidism is the result. Due to the hormonal imbalances that result, a person with hypothyroidism may experience hair loss, low energy, weight gain, exhaustion, and other issues.

The most common cause of hypothyroidism is an autoimmune condition called Hashimoto's thyroiditis or Hashimoto's disease. Because it is an inflammatory autoimmune condition, people with Hashimoto's can experience a reduction in symptoms following the paleo AIP (see page 153).

People with all types of hypothyroidism can benefit from eating foods that are rich in selenium combined with foods that are rich in iodine. Selenium-rich foods include Brazil nuts, mushrooms, brown rice, pinto beans, and sunflower seeds. Foods rich in iodine include sea vegetables, yogurt, strawberries, and cranberries, as well as iodized salt.

People with hypothyroidism may also wish to limit goitrogenic foods, which lower the production of thyroid hormones. These include cruciferous vegetables like broccoli, cabbage, radishes, and mustard, as well as soy.

IRRITABLE BOWEL SYNDROME (IBS)

For people with IBS, the continuous cycle of diarrhea, constipation, gas, and stomach pain is often debilitating and exhausting. However, recent research at Monash University in Australia has pointed to certain types of carbohydrates in foods that may be causing many of these issues. These carbohydrates are called FODMAPs, and reducing them may help improve IBS symptoms.

FODMAPs is an acronym that stands for Fermentable Oligo-Di-Monosaccharides and Polyols. These are foods that are high in fructose, such as fruit, honey, agave, and high-fructose corn syrup; lactose, which is found in dairy; fructans, which are found in onions, garlic, and wheat; galactans, which are found in legumes; and polyols, which are found in stone fruits (including avocados) and sugar alcohols like isomalt and xylitol. These foods may ferment in the intestines, leading to symptoms. Following a low-FODMAP lifestyle, however, may reduce or even eliminate symptoms associated with IBS.

INFLAMMATION

Inflammation is an immune system response against injury, illness, allergens, foreign substances, and pathogens. While it is a natural immune system response, inflammation can also be widespread, unnecessary, and even harmful. Widespread inflammation occurs in autoimmune disease, and it has been implicated as a risk factor for heart disease.

The Standard American Diet is an inflammatory diet for many reasons. Ratios of omega-6 to omega-3 essential fatty acids favor omega-6 fatty acids too heavily. Omega-6 fatty acids are necessary for the body's immune inflammatory response, but in too-high concentrations they can cause widespread inflammation. Highly processed foods contain artificial ingredients that the body may interpret as foreign invaders, responding with an inflammatory response.

To minimize unnecessary inflammation, eat a minimally processed, plant-based diet with fruits and vegetables, whole grains, nuts, seeds, fish, and poultry. Minimize artificial ingredients and sugar. Include healthy fats, such as olive oil, and eat plant and animal foods high in omega-3 fatty acids, including seafood and chia seeds.

INFLUENZA (FLU)

The flu is caused by a virus, and it can have a host of symptoms, including fever and chills, coughing, sore throat, respiratory symptoms, and diarrhea. Recent research suggests that adding selenium to the diet in the form of Brazil nuts, chia seeds, and brown rice may help prevent you from succumbing to the flu. Eating a healthy, unprocessed diet with nutrient-dense foods can help build your immune system so you are less susceptible to getting sick, even after you are exposed to bugs.

When you have the flu, it is important that you stay hydrated by drinking plenty of water, and that you meet your body's nutritional needs. Along with water, drink fruit and vegetable juices and broth to provide your body with vitamins and minerals. If you have diarrhea, follow the BRAT diet (see page 175) to sooth your stomach and help improve your stool. If you have a high fever and diarrhea, you may also want to drink unsweetened coconut water to replenish electrolytes and fluids.

INSOMNIA

Certain foods may help you get a better night's sleep, or they may lull you to sleep when nothing else will. If you ever wake up in the middle of the night with your mind racing and you can't get back to sleep, or if you never went to sleep in the first place, these nutritional solutions may be helpful.

* Don't drink alcohol before you go to bed. It disrupts REM sleep.
* Avoid drinking caffeinated beverages beyond mid-afternoon.
* Try warm milk. It has calcium in it, which induces the production of melatonin, a sleep hormone.
* Eat some yogurt or a handful of almonds before bedtime. Both contain magnesium, which has a relaxing effect on the body.
* Try some decaffeinated green tea. Green tea leaves contain the amino acid L-theanine, which has a relaxing effect.
* Eat bananas, which contain melatonin.

JOINT PAIN

Joint pain can occur as a result of autoimmune conditions like rheumatoid arthritis, or it may arise from overuse or injury. When dealing with painful, inflamed joints, eating to fight inflammation might help.

Perhaps one of the best nutritional solutions for arthritis is fish oil, which contains the omega-3 fatty acids EPA and DHA. Research shows that fish oil can reduce arthritis and joint pain. This is most likely due to the anti-inflammatory effects of the fish oil. Talk to your doctor about fish oil supplementation, and try to include fish in meals several times per week.

Avoiding inflammatory foods such as sugar, alcohol, and highly processed foods may also help. To manage inflammatory conditions such as joint pain, eat a plant-based diet full of unprocessed, nutrient-dense foods.

KIDNEY STONES

Kidney stones can be extremely painful. Depending on the size of the stone, they may move quickly through the urinary tract, or they may linger for long periods. Certain types of diets may be more conducive to the development of kidney stones, including high-protein diets. Drinking lots of caffeinated soda and not drinking enough water may also contribute to the formation of kidney stones.

One of the best ways to dislodge a kidney stone and assist it in moving quickly through the urinary tract is by drinking lots of water in a short period. Your doctor may also prescribe a medication that helps open up the urinary tract for easier passage.

People with kidney stones who wish to prevent more from forming should lower sodium in their diet. Two of the primary substances that cause kidney stones to form are oxalates and calcium. However, you don't need to avoid foods containing these substances; rather, you need to combine oxalates and calcium in the same meal. Foods that contain oxalates include dark leafy greens, berries, and almonds. Calcium-rich foods include dairy products and dark leafy greens.

Finally, some people form kidney stones from uric acid. People who form uric acid kidney stones may benefit from the recommendations for gout on page 181.

LEG CRAMPS

Leg cramps can be extremely uncomfortable, especially if they wake you up in the middle of the night. Muscle cramping can occur due to an imbalance in the electrolytes that control muscle contraction and relaxation. Leg cramps often arise as a result of a deficiency of one particular electrolyte: potassium. To relieve leg cramps, stay hydrated, even after exercise; replenish electrolytes; and eat foods high in potassium. High-potassium foods include bananas, potatoes (with the skin), sweet potatoes, and avocados. Eating foods high in other electrolytes such as calcium and magnesium may also help. Low-fat dairy products are an excellent source of both of these nutrients.

MENOPAUSE

No food or drink will stop menopause from occurring. However, eating the right foods may help with some of the more problematic symptoms of perimenopause and menopause such as hot flashes, night sweats, irritability, and other symptoms.

* To lessen the number of hot flashes you experience, Women to Women, a health clinic and website for women's health, suggests including adequate protein, healthy fats such as extra-virgin olive oil, and high-fiber plant foods in your diet.
* Since osteoporosis is more common in women past menopause, caring for bone health is essential during this time. Eat plenty of foods containing calcium, such as low-fat dairy products.
* During perimenopause, you may experience very heavy bleeding, which can lead to anemia. Eat foods high in iron and vitamin B_{12}, such as organ meats, red meat, and dark leafy greens.
* Avoid caffeine, which can increase irritability. Instead, enjoy decaffeinated green tea, which contains L-theanine for a calming effect.

MORNING SICKNESS

Morning sickness may last only a few months, but during that time it can be very uncomfortable. Despite its name, morning sickness can occur at any time throughout the day, although it is most likely to occur in the morning when you have an empty stomach.

If you have morning sickness, try eating something starchy and bland as soon as you get out of bed in the morning. Soda crackers or dry toast work well for this purpose. Continue to snack on small, bland snacks throughout the day to keep morning sickness at bay.

Some foods may help ease acute morning sickness or prevent it. Sip on ginger tea, drink ginger ale, or eat a little candied ginger for severe nausea. Squeezing lemon juice into water, or even sniffing lemons, may help clear strong nausea. Peppermint tea may also help relieve morning sickness.

OSTEOPOROSIS

Osteoporosis occurs—often in post-menopausal women—when bones become weak and brittle. When this happens, bones can easily break, so when the condition is severe enough, it can be quite painful. It is important to work with your doctor to develop strategies for improving your bone strength. In the meantime, changing your diet may also help strengthen your bones.

Regular consumption of alcoholic beverages can weaken your bones. If you have osteoporosis or are at risk for developing it, minimize your alcohol intake. Eat foods that preserve, protect, and build bone health. Include low-fat dairy products and sardines, which are an excellent source of bone-building nutrients like calcium and vitamin D. Enjoy plenty of fruits and vegetables that are high in calcium, potassium, and magnesium such as tomatoes, dark leafy greens, sweet potatoes, red peppers, oranges, and pineapples. Eat foods high in omega-3 fatty acids, which may also build bones.

PREMENSTRUAL SYNDROME (PMS)

Premenstrual syndrome encompasses a cluster of symptoms that arise due to hormonal changes in the days preceding menstruation. Symptoms may include bloating, cramps, painful breasts, and irritability, among others.

Avoid caffeine consumption, which may worsen PMS symptoms. Also, avoid excess salt, which can promote water retention, and limit sugar intake to help keep blood sugar—and mood—level.

To help with PMS-related sleep disturbances, eat bananas, which contain the sleep hormone melatonin. Vitamin B_{12}–rich foods, such as poultry, red meat, and nutritional yeast, may help boost energy levels. Meanwhile, foods rich in magnesium such as pumpkin and sesame seeds may help ease the muscle tension and cramping that is associated with PMS. Drinking plenty of water may also help with bloating, because when it is adequately hydrated your body is less likely to store excess water in the tissues.

PROSTATE ENLARGEMENT

Prostate gland enlargement happens in many men as they age. If the prostate grows too large, it may make it difficult to urinate or ejaculate. If you are experiencing symptoms of enlarged prostate, consider the following nutritional solutions:

* Minimize alcohol intake.
* Avoid caffeine.
* Don't drink anything within two hours of bedtime.
* Eat a healthy, plant-based diet that contains at least five servings of fresh produce daily.
* Choose produce in a variety of colors to ensure you are consuming an array of nutrients.
* Eat an anti-inflammatory diet that is high in omega-3 fatty acids and plant foods and low in processed foods, sugar, and red meat.
* Drink plenty of water, but spread it out evenly through the day instead of drinking several large glasses at once.

PSORIASIS

Psoriasis is an autoimmune inflammatory skin disease that causes itchy, flaking, red skin. Because it is an autoimmune disease, following the paleo (AIP, see page 153) may prevent flare-ups and may help control symptoms. As an inflammatory condition, psoriasis can also be helped by an anti-inflammatory diet that minimizes saturated fats, trans fats, red meat, caffeine, alcohol, sugar, and refined grains and includes fruits and vegetables, fish, nuts and seeds, omega-3 fatty acids, whole grains, and legumes.

Some studies have linked psoriasis to gluten consumption. Gluten is a grain found in wheat, rye, and barley, as well as oats processed in facilities where other gluten grains are processed. Gluten is present in many processed foods. Eliminating gluten may help improve psoriasis symptoms.

Losing weight may also help reduce symptoms. Eat a healthy low-calorie diet to help control weight.

ROSACEA

Rosacea is an autoimmune skin condition that results in flushed red skin, acne-like bumps, and other symptoms. Because it is an autoimmune condition, rosacea may respond to the paleo (AIP, see page 153). It may also respond to an anti-inflammatory diet of whole foods such as fruits and vegetables, whole grains, fish, poultry, and legumes.

Some foods do appear to be rosacea triggers, so these are best avoided. Rosacea trigger foods include yogurt, sour cream, cheese, soy sauce, yeast, avocados, spinach, eggplant, vinegar, spicy foods, tomatoes, citrus fruits, bananas, alcohol, caffeine, and stone fruits.

High-histamine foods may also trigger flare-ups. Foods high in histamines include fermented foods, wine, beer, foods with vinegar like pickles and mustard, and cured meats.

SINUS INFECTION/SINUSITIS

Sinusitis and sinus infections may have a number of causes, including bacteria and food sensitivities. Consuming foods to which you are sensitive or allergic (see page 195) may trigger mucous excretion in the sinus cavities, which can lead to chronic sinusitis. Determining food allergies and eliminating those foods to which you are allergic or sensitive can help relieve sinus pain and pressure.

Drinking plenty of water thins mucus and flushes out bacteria. Eating chicken soup can also thin mucus and allow it to leave your nasal passages. Spicy foods like hot mustard, chiles, and horseradish also provide a temporary clearing of nasal passages by thinning mucus and allowing it to flow. Eating garlic and onion will also help eliminate excess mucus.

SORE THROAT/LARYNGITIS

Sore throats have many causes, such as bacteria (such as strep), postnasal drip, dryness, and irritation from overuse. While sucking on a cough drop or lozenge may provide temporary relief, there are some nutritional solutions that will help as well:

* Gargle warm salt water to help shrink inflamed tissue.
* Make an alcohol-free hot toddy with warm water, honey, and lemon. The honey and lemon will soothe the throat, while the vitamin C in the lemons will provide valuable antioxidants.
* Sip warm liquids such as herbal tea or broth to soothe throat pain.
* Try a cool, bland, runny food such as a banana yogurt smoothie, which will provide nutrients without irritating your throat.

TINNITUS (RINGING IN THE EARS)

While scientific evidence is scant, anecdotal evidence from people suffering from tinnitus suggests that ringing in the ears may be made worse or exacerbated by certain foods. Triggers vary from person to person, so it's a good idea to determine your own personal triggers. Once you have determined what you think are triggers, remove those foods from your diet and then reintroduce them to see if they trigger symptoms.

Foods that may exacerbate tinnitus include excess salt, which correlates with worsening of symptoms. Caffeine and alcohol consumption may also increase symptoms.

Since tinnitus can worsen with worsening health, eating a diet that supports vibrant good health can also help minimize symptoms. Aim for a plant-based whole-foods diet high in fruits and vegetables with moderate amounts of lean proteins, whole grains, and legumes. Stay hydrated and avoid overly processed foods and sugar.

ULCERS

It was once believed that eating spicy foods caused ulcers, but current wisdom shows that most ulcers are caused by *H. pylori* bacteria. Use of alcohol and caffeine may play a role in the development of ulcers. If you have an ulcer, you may also wish to avoid foods that increase stomach acid, such as dairy products. Peppermint tea, chamomile tea, and aloe vera juice may all help soothe stomach pain associated with ulcers.

You should also pay attention to foods that trigger your pain. For example, some people may have trouble with citrus fruits, while others may not do well with tomatoes. Find your own personal triggers and remove them from your diet. If your ulcer is acting up, try eating soothing and cooling foods, such as melon, or try making a tea with ¼ teaspoon cayenne in hot water. The pepper will temporarily anesthetize the pain.

URINARY TRACT INFECTION (UTI)

Urinary tract infections can be acutely uncomfortable. The best treatment for them is prevention. To prevent urinary tract infections, drink plenty of water, avoid caffeine, and minimize sugar.

If you have a urinary tract infection, eating foods such as cranberries or blueberries will help inhibit bacterial growth in the urinary tract. Since most doctors prescribe antibiotics to treat the bacteria associated with UTIs, you'll need to replenish the healthy bacteria. To do this, eat fermented foods such as yogurt and kefir. Garlic and onions contain antimicrobial substances that may help you fight bacterial infections such as those causing UTIs. During a UTI, drink 60 to 80 ounces of water per day to flush out the urinary tract. Eating large amounts of foods high in vitamin C (or supplementing vitamin C) may help keep urine acidic, which discourages bacterial growth.

YEAST INFECTION

Yeast infections occur with yeast overgrowth. The infections can be itchy and uncomfortable. Yeast infections often occur shortly after a course of antibiotics. This happens because the antibiotics targeted at killing unhealthy bacteria also kill beneficial bacteria, allowing yeast to proliferate, which in turn can lead to yeast infection.

To control yeast infections, limit sugar in the diet and eat plenty of fermented foods, such as yogurt, kefir, and miso. These foods have active probiotic bacteria that will help recolonize and fight yeast overgrowth. Drink plenty of water and eat a healthy whole-foods diet to keep the right balance between yeast and friendly bacteria in your body so that overgrowth does not result.

food allergies

A food allergy is an immune system response to food. If you have an allergy to a certain food, your body acts abnormally, producing an antibody called immunoglobulin E (IgE).

If you are allergic to a certain food, your body produces IgE the first time you eat it, although you may not have a reaction then. Later exposures to that allergen cause symptoms to arise. Symptoms of food allergy can be mild or severe, and include itching and swelling, hives, gastrointestinal symptoms, wheezing, lowered blood pressure, throat tightening, and even a life-threatening reaction called anaphylaxis.

Food allergies are different from intolerances, which tend to be primarily digestive. Celiac disease (see page 171), for example, is an intolerance to gluten that causes stomach and intestinal issues, but it doesn't cause allergic or respiratory reactions.

A number of foods are common food allergens that affect a large percentage of the population, accounting for about 90 percent of the food allergies in the United States.

MILK AND DAIRY

Milk and dairy products are common sources of both allergies and intolerances. People who have a milk intolerance are often sensitive to the lactose in the milk, which produces gastrointestinal symptoms. People with a milk allergy tend to react to the casein in dairy products, which is a milk protein.

Milk and dairy products are the source of the most common allergies in children in the United States, affecting approximately 2.5 percent of American children under the age of three.

Because dairy products are such a good source of calcium, people with dairy allergies may wonder where they can turn to to replace calcium in their diet. Many milk substitutes, such as soymilk and almond milk, are fortified with calcium and make a suitable alternative. Calcium is also present in dark leafy greens. If you are concerned about lack of calcium due to a dairy allergy, talk with your doctor about alternatives or supplementation.

EGGS

An allergy to eggs is the second most common form of food allergy among Americans. The allergy may be mild, or it may be life-threatening. Allergies to eggs arise as a reaction to the proteins in the egg whites, called albumen. While the yolks themselves do not cause allergies, people with egg allergies should avoid both the yolks and the whites in order to avoid cross-contamination.

Eggs are contained in many processed foods and baked goods, so it is important to read labels in order to avoid accidentally ingesting eggs. Some vaccinations, such as the flu vaccination, may contain egg protein. Discuss with your doctor whether it is safe to use such vaccinations, especially in severely allergic individuals.

Egg allergies aren't just limited to chicken eggs. Instead, if you have an egg allergy, you should avoid eggs from all types of fowl, because they all contain the same protein.

PEANUTS

This common allergy can be quite severe, causing anaphylactic shock and even death. The incidence of allergies to peanuts among American children tripled in an 11-year period between 1997 and 2008. This trend doesn't seem to be unique to the United States, however. Similar statistics exist in Europe and Canada. There is no scientific evidence yet suggesting why this allergy is growing.

Even trace amounts of peanuts can trigger allergic reactions, so it is very important for parents of children who are allergic to peanuts or adults with peanut allergies to take great caution. If you or your child have a peanut allergy, read labels and avoid any foods processed in a plant that also processes peanuts or nuts. Since allergic individuals can be so sensitive, you may also need to ensure that your or your child's environment is peanut-free. Children can outgrow peanut allergies, but it is important to work closely with your doctor to make this determination.

Peanuts, by the way, are not the same as tree nuts. Rather, they are legumes.

TREE NUTS

Tree nuts are the source of another common nut allergy that can have life-threatening effects, potentially causing anaphylactic shock. About three million Americans have a tree nut allergy, some of whom also have a peanut allergy. Unlike peanut allergies, however, the rate of tree nut allergies seems to be holding fairly steady, without any statistically significant decline or growth.

Tree nuts include all types of nuts grown on trees, such as walnuts, pecans, almonds, Brazil nuts, cashews, and others. Just because you have a peanut allergy doesn't mean you're allergic to tree nuts, and just because you have a tree nut allergy does not mean you are allergic to peanuts. The two allergies are distinctly different, though they can coincide.

About 9 percent of children who have a tree nut allergy may outgrow it by the time they reach adulthood, but this should be determined by a health care professional due to the potentially life-threatening risks of ingestion.

WHEAT

Wheat is both a common allergen and a common source of food intolerance. Intolerant individuals tend to be sensitive to wheat's protein, called gluten, which can cause severe gastric issues. Some people with a gluten intolerance have the autoimmune celiac disease, while others have non-celiac gluten sensitivity. Children with wheat allergies tend to outgrow them by the time they reach adulthood. However, people with gluten sensitivity and celiac disease tend to have that intolerance their entire life.

Wheat allergies may be mild or severe. Because wheat is so ubiquitous in America's food supply, eliminating it from your diet may prove difficult but necessary. Many foods you wouldn't suspect contain wheat, such as soy sauce and mustard. Wheat may also appear on labels under other names like spelt, durum, graham, farina, triticale, couscous, emmer, and einkhorn, among others. One ingredient you don't have to worry about, however, is buckwheat, which isn't related to wheat at all and should be fine for people with wheat allergies to ingest.

SHELLFISH

People with shellfish allergies often have severe allergic reactions such as anaphylaxis. The most common type of shellfish allergy is to crustaceans, which include lobster, crab, and shrimp. Some people may also be allergic to mollusks, such as clams and oysters. In general, if you are allergic to one kind of shellfish, it is best to avoid both kinds.

Shellfish are reasonably easy to avoid, but you should always read labels so there aren't any surprises. When eating in restaurants, you need to let your server know you have a severe shellfish allergy so there is not any cross-contamination, because shellfish proteins may be airborne when cooking, landing on non-shellfish proteins. For this reason, if your allergy is severe, it is best to not eat in restaurants that primarily serve seafood.

Along with avoiding shellfish and mollusks, you need to avoid oyster sauce and fish stock, which may be made with shrimp or other crustacean shells.

FISH

Allergies to fish—such as halibut, tuna, salmon, anchovies, grouper, and other types of fish—are another common form of allergy. Fish allergies can be quite severe and may cause anaphylactic shock. Interestingly, unlike many other common allergies, a fish allergy is nearly as likely to first occur in adulthood as it is in childhood. A full 40 percent of people allergic to fish didn't experience their first reaction until they were adults. Children are unlikely to outgrow fish allergies.

Just because you are allergic to fish does not mean you are also allergic to shellfish.

SOY

Soy allergies tend to be mild to moderate, although some people have a severe reaction. The allergy can develop in infancy. Parents feeding babies soy-based formula may notice these allergies and will need to switch to non-soy infant formula. Typically, children with soy allergies outgrow them before their teenage years.

Soy products come from the soybean, which is a legume. Soy is widely used as an ingredient in processed foods, and it is also found in edamame, tempeh, tofu, soy nuts, and soy sauce. When buying processed foods, read the label carefully and watch for names of ingredients such as soy protein isolate, bean curd, hydrolyzed soy protein, miso, natto, tamari, textured vegetable protein, and teriyaki sauce.

SESAME SEEDS

While not one of the "big 8" allergies listed above, allergies to sesame seeds are growing in the United States. In the past few decades, incidence has grown steeply, although that may be due to more food offerings that contain sesame seeds.

Sesame seeds do more than pepper the outside of fast food hamburger buns. In today's cuisine, they can be found in tahini, hummus, falafel, and other Middle Eastern fare that has grown in popularity.

While sesame seed allergies can cause severe reactions such as anaphylaxis, they are more likely to cause mild to moderate symptoms such as hives, congestion, and wheezing. There may be a correlation between sesame seed allergies and tree nut allergies, so if you find that you or your children are allergic to one, you may want to check for an allergy to the other.

CELERY

Allergies to fruits and vegetables tend not to be as well-known as nut and seafood allergies, but people can develop sensitivities. One of the most common is the celery allergy. While celery doesn't need to be disclosed on American food labels, in the European Union there is enough concern about it that it must be disclosed on European food labels.

Because celery is one of the big three in aromatic vegetables that enhances the flavor of cooking (along with onions and carrots, making up a mixture called mirepoix), it's in a lot more foods than you might imagine. Celery may be used to flavor soups, stews, sauces, and chilies, so it is important to read labels or, if you are in a restaurant, talk to your server or the chef to ensure there isn't any in the food you are eating.

afterthought

I f your great-great-great grandparents saw the food you ate, would they recognize it as food? Since the mid-twentieth century, food-manufacturing processes have changed, and so has the food we eat. While the preindustrial food supply featured simple, whole ingredients like animal proteins, whole grains, fruits, vegetables, legumes, nuts, and seeds, today's supermarket offers an eye-popping array of manufactured foods that come in bags, boxes, cans, and packages. Where once the food humans ate was grown or farmed, today much of the food supply is manufactured. Many of these foods contain artificial ingredients that earlier generations never consumed.

Portion sizes have grown significantly since the middle of the 20th century, and so have waistlines. Soda drinks were once considered an occasional treat, but today Americans consume as much as 16 or 20 ounces of the fizzy beverages every day, and sometimes more. While the calories in such soft drinks meet the body's energy requirement, the beverages are entirely without nutrients. Meanwhile, fast food chains, which used to offer only one small-sized serving of French fries and sodas, now provide jumbo-sized options, and coffee shops offer 20-ounce coffee drinks loaded with fat and sugar.

As America's nutritional habits have changed and our waistlines have grown, rates of autoimmune disease, type 2 diabetes, metabolic syndrome, and other diseases associated with obesity have continued to rise. With such alarming statistics, it's clear that something is broken in the way Americans eat.

Perhaps what is needed is a return to simpler nutrition, when it wasn't necessary to read labels to know what was in your food; or, if you did, the ingredients were easily pronounced and understood. The way to health isn't through the latest and greatest low-fat and fat-free processed foods made with dozens of ingredients. It's through a return to simpler foods: whole, healthy plant foods, lean proteins, herbs, and spices.

When you eat whole, unprocessed foods, nutrition becomes simpler. If you look at one of the most successful diets in terms of heart health and weight maintenance, the Mediterranean diet does just this. It simplifies food, encouraging you to eat seasonal, locally available produce, healthful extra-virgin olive oil, flavorful herbs, a little bit of lean protein, some fish, a little bit of cheese, and occasionally some red wine. It is a diet of moderation and not excess, and it isn't based on packaged foods, but rather on simple ingredients that combine to make healthy and flavorful meals.

If you spend much time watching the news or browsing the Internet, it might seem that nutrition is extremely complex. It is easy to get caught up worrying about vitamins and minerals, balancing fatty acids, controlling calories, avoiding pesticides, and avoiding allergens and toxins. However, while knowledge is always power, there's a much simpler way to ensure you balance out all of these elements of good nutrition. Eat real food. Eat colorful food. Eat fruits and vegetables in an array of bright colors, as each color denotes different nutrients. Choose variety in your diet, and choose nutrient-dense foods instead of those with empty calories.

This is the foundation for a healthy diet: whole foods, colorful fruits and vegetables, lean proteins including fish, whole grains, low-fat dairy, legumes, nuts, and seeds. If you eat these foods most of the time, you will provide your body with the nourishment it needs to allow your health to thrive. Whenever possible, eat produce at the peak of ripeness. Enjoy seafood that has been freshly caught whenever you can. Liberally season your meals with delicious herbs and spices. And very occasionally, enjoy a sweet or sinful little something. This is the way to eat, enjoy food, and offer your body the best of the bounty nature has to offer.

how to read a nutrition label

Nutrition Facts

Serving Size 5 oz. (144g)
Servings Per Container 4

Amount Per Serving

Calories 310   **Calories** from Fat 100

                                 % Daily Value*

Total Fat 15g	**21%**
Saturated Fat 2.6g	**17%**
Trans Fat 1g	
Cholesterol 118mg	**39%**
Sodium 560mg	**28%**
Total Carbohydrate 12g	**4%**
Dietary Fiber 1g	**4%**
Sugars 1g	
Protein 24g	

Vitamin A 1%   •   **Vitamin C** 2%

Calcium 2%   •   **Iron** 5%

*Percent Daily Values are based on a 2,000 calorie diet. Your daily values may be higher or lower depending on your calorie needs:

	Calories	2,000	2,500
Total Fat	Less Than	65g	80g
Saturated Fat	Less Than	20g	25g
Cholesterol	Less Than	300mg	300mg
Sodium	Less Than	2,400mg	2,400mg
Total Carbohydrate		300g	375g
Dietary Fiber		25g	30g

Calories per gram:
  Fat 9 • Carbohydrate 4 • Protein 4

The Nutrition Facts label on processed foods supplies nutrient information according to FDA regulations. Understanding each part of the label can help you get the nutrients and calories you need daily.

Serving size: This is the amount of a single serving provided in standard sizes (cups, tablespoons, and ounces) and followed by a metric measurement (grams, etc.). A serving size might also be whole amounts, like 2 crackers or 1 container.

Servings per container: Packaged foods often have more than one serving. If you eat an entire package in one sitting that has, for example, five servings, you'll need to multiply the nutritional information by five to know how many calories and grams of fat, sodium, carbohydrates, and proteins you are consuming.

Calories: This tells you how much food energy, in calories, each serving supplies. A separate label may also tell you how many of those calories come from fat.

% Daily Value*: Sometimes shown as %DV*, this heading appears on the right-hand side of the label and refers to how much of the recommended daily amount of the nutrients in question is provided in each serving. It helps you compare similar products to see which one has higher or lower amounts of nutrients. The asterisk refers to the Percent Daily Value footnote at the bottom of the label that reminds you that the percentages of available nutrients are based on a 2,000-calorie diet.

Total Fat: "Total" refers to the total grams and total %DV of fat per serving, not per container. It includes the amounts of saturated and trans fat per serving provided beneath this listing. Monounsaturated and polyunsaturated fats may be included too, though not always listed.

Cholesterol: Cholesterol is listed per serving in milligrams (mg) with a %DV. It's important to be aware, however, that available evidence shows that trans fats have a stronger link to blood cholesterol than dietary cholesterol does.

Sodium: Sodium is listed per serving and in milligrams (mg) with a %DV. One teaspoon of sodium (2,300 mg) is recommended per day.

Total Carbohydrates: "Total" refers to the total grams and total %DV of carbohydrates per *serving*, not per container. It includes the amount of fiber and sugar per serving given beneath this listing. "Other carbohydrates," which can refer to starches and/or sugar alcohols (reduced-calorie sweeteners), can also be included, though they may not be listed.

Protein: Protein is listed per serving in grams, and lists a %DV only if the product is meant for children younger than four or is claimed to be high in protein.

Vitamins and minerals: The %DV for vitamins A and C, calcium, and iron must be listed here along with other vitamins or minerals that have been added to the food.

Ingredients: All the ingredients used to make the food are included here. They are listed by weight, from the most to the least. This means that the product contains more of the first few ingredients than the last ingredients listed.

conversions

VOLUME EQUIVALENTS (LIQUID)

US STANDARD	US STANDARD (OUNCES)	METRIC (APPROXIMATE)
2 tablespoons	1 fl. oz.	30 mL
¼ cup	2 fl. oz.	60 mL
½ cup	4 fl. oz.	120 mL
1 cup	8 fl. oz.	240 mL
1½ cups	12 fl. oz.	355 mL
2 cups or 1 pint	16 fl. oz.	475 mL
4 cups or 1 quart	32 fl. oz.	1 L
1 gallon	128 fl. oz.	4 L

OVEN TEMPERATURES

FAHRENHEIT (F)	CELSIUS (C) (APPROXIMATE)
250°	120°
300°	150°
325°	165°
350°	180°
375°	190°
400°	200°
425°	220°
450°	230°

VOLUME EQUIVALENTS (DRY)

US STANDARD	METRIC (APPROXIMATE)
⅛ teaspoon	0.5 mL
¼ teaspoon	1 mL
½ teaspoon	2 mL
¾ teaspoon	4 mL
1 teaspoon	5 mL
1 tablespoon	15 mL
¼ cup	59 mL
⅓ cup	79 mL
½ cup	118 mL
⅔ cup	156 mL
¾ cup	177 mL
1 cup	235 mL
2 cups or 1 pint	475 mL
3 cups	700 mL
4 cups or 1 quart	1 L

WEIGHT EQUIVALENTS

US STANDARD	METRIC (APPROXIMATE)
½ ounce	15 g
1 ounce	30 g
2 ounces	60 g
4 ounces	115 g
8 ounces	225 g
12 ounces	340 g
16 ounces or 1 pound	455 g

references

INTRODUCTION

"An Epidemic of Obesity: U.S. Obesity Trends." *The Nutrition Source*. Accessed May 7, 2015. www.hsph.harvard.edu /nutritionsource/an-epidemic-of-obesity/.

"Adult Obesity Facts." Centers for Disease Control and Prevention, Sept. 9, 2014. www.cdc.gov/obesity/data/adult.html.

"National Cardiovascular Disease Surveillance." Centers for Disease Control and Prevention, May 7, 2014. www.cdc.gov /dhdsp/ncvdss/index.htm.

Autoimmune Diseases Research Plan. Bethesda, MD: National Institutes of Health, 2002. U.S. Department of Health and Human Services. www.niaid.nih.gov/topics/autoimmune /documents/adccreport.pdf.

CHAPTER ONE: NUTRITION & HEALTH

"Nutrition and the Health of Young People." Centers for Disease Control and Prevention, Oct. 6, 2014. www.cdc.gov/healthyyouth /nutrition/facts.htm.

WHAT NUTRITION IS

"Nutrition." World Health Organization. Accessed May 7, 2015. www.who.int/topics/nutrition/en/.

Macronutrients: The Importance of Carbohydrate, Protein, and Fat." McKinley Health Center, University of Illinois. Accessed May 7, 2015. www.mckinley.illinois.edu/handouts /macronutrients.htm.

"Micronutrients." World Health Organization. Accessed May 7, 2015. www.who.int/nutrition/topics/micronutrients/en/.

WHAT NUTRITION ISN'T

Heneman, Karrie, and Sheri Zidenberg-Cherr. *Nutrition and Health Info-Sheet*. October 2008. Department of Nutrition, UC Davis. www.nutrition.ucdavis.edu/content/infosheets /fact-pro-phytochemical.pdf.

Corliss, Julie. "Eating Too Much Added Sugar Increases the Risk of Dying with Heart Disease." Harvard Health Blog. Feb. 6, 2014. www.health.harvard.edu/blog/eating-too-much-added-sugar -increases-the-risk-of-dying-with-heart-disease-201402067021.

HISTORICAL FACTS AND TRIVIA

"Lincoln's Agricultural Legacy." USDA National Agricultural Library. Accessed May 7, 2015. www.nal.usda.gov/lincolns -agricultural-legacy.

"FSIS History." USDA. Accessed May 7, 2015. www.fsis.usda.gov /wps/portal/informational/aboutfsis/history/history.

Yang, Quanhe, Zefeng Zhang, Edward W. Gregg, Dana Flanders, et al. "Sugar Intake and Cardiovascular Diseases Mortality." JAMA Network. *JAMA Internal Medicine*. Accessed May 7, 2015. www.archinte.jamanetwork.com/article.aspx?articleid=1819573.

"FDA History—Part I." U.S. Food and Drug Administration. Accessed May 7, 2015. www.fda.gov/AboutFDA/WhatWeDo /History/Origin/ucm054819.htm.

"Meat Inspection Act of 1906—United States [1906]." *Encyclopedia Britannica Online*, accessed May 7, 2015. www.britannica. com/EBchecked/topic/371753/Meat-Inspection-Act-of-1906.

"Ancel Keys and the Lipid Hypothesis: From Early Breakthroughs to Current Management of Dyslipidemia." *BC Medical Journal*. Accessed May 7, 2015. www.bcmj.org/article/ancel-keys-and -lipid-hypothesis-early-breakthroughs-current-management -dyslipidemia.

"Vitamin B$_{12}$." University of Maryland Medical Center. Accessed May 7, 2015. www.umm.edu/health/medical/ency/articles /vitamin-b12.

"USDA Profiling Food Consumption in America." *Agriculture Fact Book, 2001–2002*, 13–21. Accessed May 7, 2015. www.usda.gov /factbook/chapter2.pdf.

Weil, Andrew. "Balanced Living." Accessed May 7, 2015. www.drweil.com/drw/u/ART02837/ten-surprising-nutrition -facts-from-Dr-Weil.html.

Center for Food Safety. Accessed May 7, 2015. www.centerfor-foodsafety.org/issues/311/ge-foods/about-ge-foods.

HOW NUTRITION RELATES TO GROWTH, REPRODUCTION, HEALTH, METABOLISM

Walker, A. R. P., B. F. Walker, and John Dobbing. "Fetal Nutrition and Cardiovascular Disease in Adult Life." *The Lancet* 341.8857 (1993): 1421–22.

"Neural Tube Defects: MedlinePlus." U.S. National Library of Medicine. Accessed May 7, 2015. www.nlm.nih.gov/medlineplus /neuraltubedefects.html.

Chase, H. Peter, and Harold P. Martin. "Undernutrition and Child Development." *New England Journal of Medicine* 282.17 (1970): 933–39.

Jukes, Matthew, Judity McGuire, Frank Method, and Robert Sternberg. "Nutrition and Education." *Nutrition: A Foundation for Education*. Accessed May 7, 2015. www.unscn.org/files /Publications/Briefs_on_Nutrition/Brief2_Edf.

"Nutrition and Reproduction in Women." *Human Reproduction Update* 12.3 (2006): 193–207.

Van Der Spuy, Z. M. "Nutrition and Reproduction." Clinics in Obstetrics and Gynaecology. Accessed May 7, 2015. www.europepmc.org/abstract/med/3905160.

"Dietary Reference Intakes." USDA National Agricultural Library. Accessed May 7, 2015. www.fnic.nal.usda.gov/dietary -guidance/dietary-reference-intakes.

"Scurvy: MedlinePlus Medical Encyclopedia." U.S. National Library of Medicine. Accessed May 7, 2015. www.nlm.nih.gov /medlineplus/ency/article/000355.htm.

"Rickets: MedlinePlus Medical Encyclopedia." U.S. National Library of Medicine. Accessed May 7, 2015. www.nlm.nih.gov /medlineplus/ency/article/000344.htm.

WHAT "HEALTHY" MEANS

"WHO Definition of Health." Accessed May 7, 2015. www.who.int /about/definition/en/print.html.

"Celiac Disease." National Center for Biotechnology Information. U.S. National Library of Medicine. Accessed May 7, 2015. www.ncbi.nlm.nih.gov/pubmedhealth/PMHT0024528/.

FOOD AS MEDICINE

"The Low-FODMAP Diet." Stanford University. Accessed May 7, 2015. www.stanfordhealthcare.org/content/dam/SHC /for-patients-component/programs-services/clinical-nutrition -services/docs/pdf-lowfodmapdiet.pdf.

"Examples of Traditional Fermented Foods That Boost Digestive Health." *Dr. David Williams* (blog). Accessed May 7, 2015. www.drdavidwilliams.com/digestive-health-fermented -foods-main/.

"Iron Deficiency—Anemia." Mayo Clinic. Accessed May 7, 2015. www.mayoclinic.org/diseases-conditions/iron-deficiency -anemia/basics/prevention/con-20019327.

"Vitamin C and Colds: MedlinePlus Medical Encyclopedia." U.S. National Library of Medicine. Accessed May 7, 2015. www.nlm.nih.gov/medlineplus/ency/article/002145.htm.

FOOD WITH MEDICINE, FOOD VERSUS MEDICINE

"Avoid Food and Drug Interactions." U.S. Food and Drug Administration 106.20 (1974): 312. Accessed May 7, 2015. www.fda.gov /downloads/Drugs/ResourcesForYou/Consumers /BuyingUsingMedicineSafely/EnsuringSafeUseofMedicine /GeneralUseofMedicine/UCM229033.pdf.

"High Cholesterol." Mayo Clinic. Accessed May 7, 2015. www.mayoclinic.org/diseases-conditions/high-blood-cholesterol/in-depth/niacin/art-20046208.

Simopoulos, Artemis P. "Omega-3 Fatty Acids in Inflammation and Autoimmune Diseases." *Journal of the American College of Nutrition* 21.6 (2002): 495–505.

ADDITIONAL REFERENCES

"Who, What, Why: Can Foods Have Negative Calories?" BBC News. Accessed May 7, 2015. www.bbc.com/news/magazine-21723312.

Rohers, Timothy, and Thomas Roth. "Sleep, Sleepiness, and Alcohol Use." NIH National Institute on Alcoholism and Alcohol Abuse. National Institutes of Health. Accessed May 7, 2015. www.pubs.niaaa.nih.gov/publications/arh25-2/101-109.htm.

"Eggs: Are They Good or Bad for My Cholesterol?" Mayo Clinic. Accessed May 7, 2015. www.mayoclinic.org/diseases-conditions/high-blood-cholesterol/expert-answers/cholesterol/faq-20058468.

Subramian, Sushma. "Fact or Fiction: Raw Veggies Are Healthier than Cooked Ones." *Scientific American.* Accessed May 7, 2015. www.scientificamerican.com/article/raw-veggies-are-healthier/.

Simopoulos, A. P. "The Importance of the Ratio of Omega-6/Omega-3 Essential Fatty Acids." *Biomedicine & Pharmacotherapy* 56.8 (2002): 365–79.

CHAPTER TWO: THE BODY

DIGESTION, ABSORPTION, METABOLISM

"Your Digestive System and How It Works." National Institutes of Health. Accessed May 7, 2015. www.niddk.nih.gov/health-information/health-topics/anatomy/your-digestive-system/Pages/anatomy.aspx.

"Your Digestive System." KidsHealth. Ed. Yamini Durani. The Nemours Foundation, Oct. 1, 2012. www.kidshealth.org/kid/htbw/digestive_system.html.

"How the Small Intestine Works." Seattle Children's Hospital. Accessed May 7, 2015. www.seattlechildrens.org/clinics-programs/transplant/intestine/how-the-small-intestine-works/.

"Gross and Microscopic Anatomy of the Small Intestine." Colorado State University. Accessed May 7, 2015. www.vivo.colostate.edu/hbooks/pathphys/digestion/smallgut/anatomy.html.

"The Small Intestine: Introduction and Index." Colorado State University. Accessed May 7, 2015. www.vivo.colostate.edu/hbooks/pathphys/digestion/smallgut/index.html.

"Absorption in the Small Intestine: General Mechanisms." Colorado State University. Accessed May 7, 2015. www.vivo.colostate.edu/hbooks/pathphys/digestion/smallgut/absorb.html.

"Metabolism." MedlinePlus Medical Encyclopedia. U.S. National Library of Medicine. Accessed May 7, 2015. www.nlm.nih.gov/medlineplus/ency/article/002257.htm.

"Metabolism." KidsHealth. Ed. Steven Dowshen. The Nemours Foundation, Feb. 1, 2012. www.kidshealth.org/teen/your_body/body_basics/metabolism.html.

NOURISHING THE BODY

"Why Does the Brain Need So Much Power?" *Scientific American.* Accessed May 7, 2015. www.scientificamerican.com/article/why-does-the-brain-need-s/.

Jabr, Ferris. "Does Thinking Really Hard Burn More Calories?" *Scientific American.* Accessed May 7, 2015. www.scientificamerican.com/article/thinking-hard-calories/.

"Neuroscience for Kids—Nutrition and the Brain." Accessed May 7, 2015. www.faculty.washington.edu/chudler/nutr.html.

Perlmutter, David. "Your Brain Needs Cholesterol." Accessed May 7, 2015. www.drperlmutter.com/brain-needs-cholesterol/.

West, Rebecca, Michal Schnaider Beeri, James Schmeidler, Christine M. Hannigan, et al. "Better Memory Functioning Associated With Higher Total and Low-Density Lipoprotein Cholesterol Levels in Very Elderly Subjects Without the Apolipoprotein E4 Allele." *American Journal of Geriatric Psychiatry* 16:9 (2008), 781–85.

"About Cholesterol." American Heart Association. Accessed May 8, 2015. www.heart.org/HEARTORG/Conditions/Cholesterol/AboutCholesterol/About-Cholesterol_UCM_001220_Article.jsp.

"Neuroscience: Low Vitamin E Levels Can Affect Brain Health." *International Business Times*, Apr. 14, 2015. www.ibtimes.co.uk/neuroscience-low-vitamin-e-levels-can-affect-brain-health-1496254.

Gómez-Pinilla, Fernando. "Brain Foods: The Effects of Nutrients on Brain Function." *Nature Reviews Neuroscience* 9:7 (2008), 568–78.

Maron, Dina Fine. "Fact or Fiction? Carrots Improve Your Vision." *Scientific American*. Accessed May 7, 2015. www.scientificamerican.com/article/fact-or-fiction-carrots-improve-your-vision/.

Gomez-Pinilla, Fernando. "Diet & Nutrition." *National Review of Neuroscience*, July 28, 2009. www.aoa.org/patients-and-public/caring-for-your-vision/diet-and-nutrition?sso=y.

"Caring for Your Vision." *Diet & Nutrition*. Accessed May 7, 2015. www.aoa.org/patients-and-public/caring-for-your-vision/diet-and-nutrition?sso=y.

Spankovich, C., and C. G. Le Prell. "Healthy Diets, Healthy Hearing: National Health and Nutrition Examination Survey, 1999–2002." *International Journal of Audiology* 52.6 (2013): 369–76.

"Nutrition." American Dental Association. Accessed May 7, 2015. www.mouthhealthy.org/en/nutrition/.

"Micronutrients and Skin Health." Linus Pauling Institute. Oregon State University. Accessed May 7, 2015. www.lpi.oregonstate.edu/mic/micronutrients-health/skin-health

Richer, Stuart, William Stiles, Laisvyde Statkute, Jose Pulido, et al. "Double-Masked, Placebo-Controlled, Randomized Trial of Lutein and Antioxidant Supplementation in the Intervention of Atrophic Age-Related Macular Degeneration: The Veterans LAST Study (Lutein Antioxidant Supplementation Trial)." *Optometry—Journal of the American Optometric Association* 75:4 (2004), 216–29.

"Vitamin C." America Optometric Association, accessed May 7, 2015. www.aoa.org/patients-and-public/caring-for-your-vision/diet-and-nutrition/vitamin-c?sso=y.

"Essential Fatty Acids." American Optometric Association. Accessed May 7, 2015. www.aoa.org/patients-and-public/caring-for-your-vision/diet-and-nutrition/essential-fatty-acids?sso=y.

"Zinc." American Optometric Association. Accessed May 7, 2015. www.aoa.org/patients-and-public/caring-for-your-vision/diet-and-nutrition/zinc?sso=y.

"The American Heart Association's Diet and Lifestyle Recommendations." American Heart Association. Accessed May 7, 2015. www.heart.org/HEARTORG/GettingHealthy/NutritionCenter/HealthyEating/The-American-Heart-Associations-Diet-and-Lifestyle-Recommendations_UCM_305855_Article.jsp.

"Vitamin and Mineral Supplements." American Heart Association. Accessed May 7, 2015. www.heart.org/HEARTORG/GettingHealthy/NutritionCenter/Vitamin-and-Mineral-Supplements_UCM_306033_Article.jsp.

"Nutrition." American Lung Association. Accessed May 7, 2015. www.lung.org/lung-disease/copd/living-with-copd/nutrition.html.

Romieu, I. "Nutrition and Lung Health." *International Journal of Tuberculosis and Lung Disease* 9:04 (2005), n. pag. Accessed May 7, 2015. www.ncbi.hih.gov/pubmed/1583074.

"Breast Cancer Statistics." Centers for Disease Control and Prevention, Sept. 2, 2014. www.cdc.gov/cancer/breast/statistics/.

"Basic Facts About Breast Health: Nutrition for Breast Cancer Prevention." University of California, San Francisco. Accessed May 7, 2015. www.ucsfhealth.org/education/breast_health/nutrition_for_breast_cancer_prevention/.

Ketteler, Judi. "Back Pain—The Healthy Back Diet." The Cleveland Clinic, June 3, 2010. www.clevelandclinicwellness.com/conditions/BackPain/Pages/TheHealthyBackDiet.aspx#.

"Blood Basics." American Society of Hematology. Accessed May 7, 2015. www.hematology.org/Patients/Basics/.

"Calcium, Nutrition, and Bone Health." American Academy of Orthopedic Surgeons. Accessed May 8, 2015. www.orthoinfo.aaos.org/topic.cfm?topic=A00317.

"Iron-Deficiency Anemia." American Society of Hematology. Accessed May 8, 2015. www.hematology.org/patients/blood-donation/deficiencies.php.

"Neuroscience for Kids—Nutrition and the Brain." University of Washington. Accessed May 8, 2015. www.faculty.washington.edu/chudler/nutr2.html.

Yung, Kwon sub, and Len Kravitz. "How Do Muscles Grow?" University of New Mexico. Accessed May 8, 2015. www.unm.edu/~lkravitz/Article%20folder/musclesgrowLK.html.

"Endocrine Glands and Types of Hormones." Hormone Health Network. Accessed May 8, 2015. www.hormone.org/hormones-and-health/the-endocrine-system/endocrine-glands-and-types-of-hormones.

Bikle, D. D. "The Vitamin D Endocrine System." *Advanced Internal Medicine* 27 (1982): 45–71.

Abercrombie, Jennifer. "Balancing the Endocrine System Naturally." Naturopathic Wellness Center, Mar. 6, 2012. www.nawellness.com/balancing-the-endocrine-system-naturally/.

Pick, Marcelle. "Goitrogens and Thyroid Health." Women to Women. Accessed May 8, 2015. www.womentowomen.com/thyroid-health/goitrogens-and-thyroid-health-the-good-news/.

"Your Urinary System." KidsHealth. Ed. Rupal Christine Gupta. The Nemours Foundation, Sept. 1, 2014. www.kidshealth.org/kid/htbw/pee.html.

"The DASH Diet." National Kidney Foundation. Accessed May 8, 2015. www.kidney.org/atoz/content/Dash_Diet.

"Your Digestive System and How It Works." National Institute of Diabetes and Digestive and Kidney Diseases. Accessed May 8, 2015. www.niddk.nih.gov/health-information/health-topics/Anatomy/your-digestive-system/Pages/anatomy.aspx.

Scarlata, Kate. *Low-FODMAP 28-Day Plan: A Healthy Cookbook with Gut-Friendly Recipes for IBS Relief.* Berkeley, CA: Rockridge, 2014.

NOURISHING THE MIND

"The Human Brain—Carbohydrates." The Franklin Institute. Accessed May 8, 2015. www.learn.fi.edu/learn/brain/carbs.html.

"Cells of the Nervous System." University of Washington. Accessed May 8, 2015. www.faculty.washington.edu/chudler/cells.html.

"Nourish—Carbohydrates Fuel Your Brain." The Franklin Institute. Accessed May 8, 2015. www.learn.fi.edu/learn/brain/proteins.html.

"The Human Brain—Fats." The Franklin Institute. Accessed May 8, 2015. www.learn.fi.edu/learn/brain/fats.html.

"High Good and Low Bad Cholesterol Levels Are Healthy for the Brain, Too." University of California, Davis, Dec. 30, 2013. Accessed May 8, 2015. www.ucdmc.ucdavis.edu/publish/news/newsroom/8555.

"Flavonoids: The Diet's Effect on Human Memory and Learning." Royal Society of Chemistry, Feb. 26, 2009. www.rsc.org/Publishing/Journals/cb/Volume/2009/4/Food_for_thought.asp.

Selhub, Jacob, Aron Troen, and Irwin H. Rosenberg. "B Vitamins and the Aging Brain." *Nutrition Reviews* 68 (2010): S112–18.

"Information on the Latest Vitamin D News and Research." Vitamin D Council. Accessed May 8, 2015. www.vitamindcouncil.org/health-conditions/cognitive-impairment/.

Harrison, Fiona E., and James M. May. "Vitamin C Function in the Brain: Vital Role of the Ascorbate Transporter (SVCT2)." *Free Radical Biology & Medicine* (March 15, 2009) 46(6): 719–30. Accessed May 8, 2015. www.ncbi.nlm.nih.gov/pmc/articles/PMC2649700/.

"Vitamin C Function in the Brain: Vital Role of the Ascorbate Transporter (SVCT2)." Micronutrient Information Center. Linus Pauling Institute, Oregon State University. Accessed May 8, 2015. www.lpi.oregonstate.edu/mic/vitamins/vitamin-C.

Zeisel, Steven H. "Nutritional Importance of Choline for Brain Development." *Journal of the American College of Nutrition* 23.Sup6 (2004): 621S–26S.

Grodstein, F., J. H. Kang, R. J. Glynn, N. R. Cook, and J. M. Gaziano. "A Randomized Trial of Beta Carotene Supplementation and Cognitive Function in Men: The Physicians' Health Study II." *Archives of Internal Medicine* 167.20 (2007): 2184–190.

Whanger, P. D. "Selenium and the Brain: A Review." *Nutritional Neuroscience* 4.2 (2001): 81–97.

"Calcium and Alzheimer's Disease." The Green Lab. University of California, Irvine, accessed May 8, 2015. www.faculty.sites.uci.edu/kimgreen/bio/calcium-and-alzheimers-disease/.

Yarlagadda, Atmaram, Shaifali Kaushik, and Anita H. Clayton. "Blood Brain Barrier: The Role of Calcium Homeostasis." *Psychiatry* (December 4, 2007) 4 (12): 55-59. www.ncbi.nlm.nih.gov/pmc/articles/PMC2861516/.

Pfeiffer, C. C., and E. R. Braverman. "Zinc, the Brain, and Behavior." *Biological Psychiatry* 17.4 (1982): 513–32.

Pinero, Domingo J., and James R. Connor. "Iron in the Brain: An Important Contributor in Normal and Diseased States." *Neuroscientist.* Accessed May 8, 2015. www.nro.sagepub.com/content/6/6/435.abstract.

Yarris, Lynn. "Copper on the Brain at Rest." Berkeley Lab, Nov. 26, 2014. www.newscenter.lbl.gov/2014/11/26/copper-on-the-brain-at-rest/.

ADDITIONAL REFERENCES

Ruth S. Macdonald, " The Role of Zinc in Growth and Cell Proliferation, "*The Journal of Nutrition* vol. 130, no. 5 (May 1, 2000), 1500S-1508S. www.jn.nutrition.org/content/130/5/1500S.

CHAPTER THREE: NUTRIENTS

MACRONUTRIENTS: CARBOHYDRATES, FATS, AND PROTEINS

"What Is Carbohydrate Deficiency?" The University of Chicago Celiac Disease Center. Accessed March 23, 2015. www.cureceliacdisease.org/archives/faq/what-is-carbohydrate-deficiency.

"Dietary Reference Intakes DRIs." Institute of Medicine, National Academy of Sciences. Accessed May 20, 2015. www.nal.usda.gov/fnic/DRI/DRI_Energy/energy_full_report.pdf.

"Dietary Guidelines for Americans, 2015." Health.gov. www.health.gov/dietaryguidelines/2015.asp

Bilsborough, S., and N. Mann. "A Review of Issues of Dietary Protein Intake in Humans." *International Journal of Sport Nutrition and Exercise Metabolism* 16:2 (Apr. 2006), 129–52.

MICRONUTRIENTS: VITAMINS, MINERALS, AND WATER

"Vitamin B5 (Pantothenic Acid)." University of Maryland. Accessed May 20, 2015. www. umm.edu/health/medical/altmed/supplement/vitamin-b5-pantothenic-acid

"Vitamin B6 (Pyridoxine)." University of Maryland. Accessed May 20, 2015. www.umm.edu/health/medical/altmed/supplement/vitamin-b5-pantothenic-acid

"Vitamin D: Fact Sheet for Health Professionals." National Institutes of Health. Accessed May 20, 2015. www.ods.od.nih.gov/factsheets/VitaminD-HealthProfessional/

"Vitamin E: Fact Sheet for Health Professionals." National Institutes of Health. Accessed May 20, 2015. www.ods.od.nih.gov/factsheets/VitaminE-HealthProfessional/

Omudhome Ogbru. "Bismuth Subsalicylate (Pepto Bismol, Kaopectate, Bismatrol Maximum Strength, and Others)." MedicineNet.com. Accessed May 20, 2015. www.medicinenet.com/bismuth_subsalicylate-oral/page2.htm.

Ross, A. C., C. L. Taylor, A. L. Yaktine, and H. B. Del Valle, editors. "Dietary Reference Intakes for Calcium and Vitamin D." Institute of Medicine (US). Washington, DC: National Academies Press, 2011. www.ncbi.nlm.nih.gov/books/NBK56070/.

Meletis, Chris. "Chloride: The Forgotten Essential Mineral." Trace Minerals Research. Accessed May 21, 2015. www.traceminerals.com/research/chloride.

"Chromium: Dietary Supplement Fact Sheet." National Institutes of Health. Accessed May 21, 2015. www.ods.od.nih.gov/factsheets/Chromium-HealthProfessional/.

"Copper." Linus Pauling Institute. Oregon State University. Accessed May 21, 2015. www.lpi.oregonstate.edu/mic/minerals/copper.

"Hyponatremia." Mayo Clinic. Accessed May 8, 2015. www.mayoclinic.org/diseases-conditions/hyponatremia/expert-answers/low-blood-sodium/faq-20058465.

Margen, Sheldon. *Wellness Foods A to Z: An Indispensable Guide for Health-Conscious Food Lovers*, editors John Swartzberg and U.C. Berkeley Wellness Letter Staff. Berkeley, CA: University Health Publishing, 2002.

"Zinc: Fact Sheet for Health Professionals." Office of Dietary Supplements. National Institutes of Health, June 5, 2013. www.ods.od.nih.gov/factsheets/Zinc-HealthProfessional/.

"Zinc." Linus Pauling Institute, Oregon State University. Accessed July 13 2015. www.lpi.oregonstate.edu/mic/minerals/zinc.

"Zinc in Diet." MedlinePlus. U.S. National Library of Medicine. Feb 2, 2013. www.nlm.nih.gov/medlineplus/ency/article/002416.htm.

Rink, Lothar. and Philip Gabriel. "Zinc and the Immune System." *Proceedings of Nutrition Society* 59:4 (Nov 2000), 541–52.

Caldwell, Emily. "Zinc Helps Against Infection by Tapping Brakes in Immune Response." Research and Innovation Communications. Ohio State University. Accessed July 13, 2015. www.researchnews.osu.edu/archive/zip8.htm.

Pfeiffer, C.C., and E.R. Braverman. "Zinc, the Brain and Behavior." *Biological Psychaiatry* 12.4 (Apr 1982).

MacDonald. R.S., "The Role of Zinc in Growth and Cell Proliferation." *Journal of Nutrition* 130.5S Suppl. (May 2000), 1500S–8S.

ADDITIONAL REFERENCES

Osler, M. "The Food Intake of Smokers and Nonsmokers: The Role of Partner's Smoking Behavior," *Preventive Medicine* 27:3 (May–June 1998), 438–43. www.ncbi.nlm.nih.gov/pubmed/9612834.

"Heart-Healthy Cooking: Oils 101." Cleveland Clinic, Oct. 1, 2014. www.health.clevelandclinic.org/2014/10/heart-healthy-cooking-oils-101/.

CHAPTER FOUR: EATING

FOOD

"Dietary Fats: Know which Types to Choose." Nutrition and Healthy Eating. Mayo Clinic. Accessed May 8, 2015. www.mayoclinic.org/healthy-lifestyle/nutrition-and-healthy-eating/in-depth/fat/art-20045550.

"Meat and Poultry Labeling Terms." USDA. Accessed May 8, 2015. www.fsis.usda.gov/wps/portal/fsis/topics/food-safety-education/get-answers/food-safety-fact-sheets/food-labeling/meat-and-poultry-labeling-terms/meat-and-poultry-labeling-terms.

"Where's the Better Beef?" National Resources Defense Council. Accessed May 8, 2015. www.nrdc.org/food/better-beef-production/.

Mankad, Rekha. "Does Grass-Fed Beef Have Any Heart-Health Benefits That Other Types of Beef Don't?" Mayo Clinic. Accessed May 8, 2015. www.us-mg4.mail.yahoo.com/neo/launch?.partner=sbc&.rand=25k2ie91q8uf1#.

"Health Benefits of Meats, Beans, and Nuts." HealthyEating.org. Dairy Council of California. Accessed May 8, 2015. www.healthyeating.org/Healthy-Eating/All-Star-Foods/Meat-Beans.aspx.

Masterjohn, Christopher. "Fatty Acid Analysis of Grass-Fed and Grain-Fed Beef Tallow." The Weston A. Price Foundation, Jan. 21, 2014. www.westonaprice.org/health-topics/fatty-acid-analysis -of-grass-fed-and-grain-fed-beef-tallow/.

"Protein." Centers for Disease Control and Prevention, Oct. 4, 2012. www.cdc.gov/nutrition/everyone/basics/protein.html.

"Fats and Cholesterol: Out with the Bad, In with the Good." Harvard School of Public Health. Accessed May 8, 2015. www.hsph .harvard.edu/nutritionsource/fats-full-story/.

Teicholz, Nina. *The Big Fat Surprise: Why Butter, Meat, and Cheese Belong in a Healthy Diet*. New York: Simon & Schuster, 2015.

Minger, Denise. *Death by Food Pyramid*. Malibu, CA: Primal Nutrition, 2014.

Weil, Andrew. "Q & A Library: Organ Meats: Liver Lover?" *Dr. Andrew Weil* (blog). Accessed May 8, 2015. www.drweil.com /drw/u/QAA401116/Organ-Meats-Liver-Lover.html.

"How Much Food from the Dairy Group is Needed Daily?" Choose My Plate.gov. USDA. Accessed May 8, 2015. www. choosemyplate .gov/food-groups/dairy-amount.html.

"Milk Protein." Milk Facts. Accessed May 8, 2015. www.milkfacts .info/Milk%20Composition/Protein.htm.

"What Is Casein? Foods with Casein, Casein Allergies, and More." WebMD. Accessed May 8, 2015. www.webmd.com/allergies /guide/casein-allergy-overview?page=3.

Månsson, Helena Lindmark. "Fatty Acids in Bovine Milk Fat." *Food and Nutrition Research*. (June 2008) 52 doi:103402 /frn.v52i0.1821. www.ncbi.nlm.nih.gov/pmc/articles /PMC2596709/.

"Nutrients in Milk; Health Benefits of Milk; Nutrients in Different Types of Milk; Sugar in Milk." HealthyEating.org. California Dairy Council. Accessed May 8, 2015. www.healthyeating.org /Milk-Dairy/Nutrients-in-Milk-Cheese-Yogurt/Nutrients-in -Milk.aspx.

Spiegel, Alison. "Pasteurized vs. Homogenized Milk: What's the Difference?" TheHuffingtonPost.com, July 22, 2014. www.huffingtonpost.com/2014/07/22/pasteurized-homogenized -milk_n_5606168.html.

"Nutriton Claims for Dairy Products." Dairy Research Institute. Accessed May 8, 2015. www.usdairy.com/~/media/usd/public /quick-reference%20guide.pdf.pdf

"Seafood Health Facts: Making Smart Choices." USDA. Accessed May 8, 2015. www. seafoodhealthfacts.org/pdf/seafood-nutrition -hp-nutrient-chart.pdf.

"Fish and Omega-3 Fatty Acids." American Heart Association. Accessed May 8, 2015. www.heart.org/HEARTORG /GettingHealthy/NutritionCenter/HealthyDietGoals/Fish-and -Omega-3-Fatty-Acids_UCM_303248_Article.jsp.

"Healing Foods Pyramid." The University of Michigan Health System. Accessed May 8, 2015. www.med.umich.edu/umim /food-pyramid/fish.html.

"Mercury Levels in Fish." NDRC. Accessed May 8, 2015. www.nrdc.org/health/effects/mercury/guide.asp.

"What You Need to Know about Mercury in Fish and Shellfish." Water Outreach & Communication. Environmental Protection Agency, 2004. www.water.epa.gov/scitech/swguidance /fishshellfish/outreach/advice_index.cfm.

"Guidance for Industry: The Seafood List." FDA. Accessed May 8, 2015. www.fda.gov/Food/GuidanceRegulation /GuidanceDocumentsRegulatoryInformation/Seafood/ ucm113260.htm.

"Seafood Labels." Food & Water Watch. Accessed May 8, 2015. www.foodandwaterwatch.org/common-resources/fish/seafood /labeling/.

"Farmed Salmon vs. Wild Salmon." Washington State Department of Health. Accessed May 8, 2015. www.doh.wa.gov /CommunityandEnvironment/Food/Fish/FarmedSalmon.

Oaklander, Mandy. "Which Is Healthier: Wild Salmon vs. Farmed Salmon." *Prevention*. Accessed May 8, 2015. www.prevention.com /content/which-healthier-wild-salmon-vs-farmed-salmon.

"Seafood and Nutrition." Oregon State University. Accessed May 8, 2015. www.seafoodhealthfacts.org/seafood_nutrition /practitioners/seafood_nutrition_overview.php.

"Fruits and Vegetables." K-State Research and Extension. Accessed May 8, 2015. www.ksre.k-state.edu/HumanNutrition /~/doc11619.ashx

"Eating Healthy with Cruciferous Vegetables." World's Healthiest Foods. Accessed May 8, 2015. www.whfoods.com/genpage .php?tname=btnews&dbid=126.

Busch, Sandy. "Nightshade Family Nutrition." *SF Gate*. Accessed May 8, 2015. www.healthyeating.sfgate.com/nightshade-family -nutrition-2878.html.

"Green Beans." World's Healthiest Foods. Accessed May 8, 2015. www.whfoods.com/genpage.php?tname=foodspice&dbid=134.

"Mushrooms, Crimini." World's Healthiest Foods. Accessed May 8, 2015. www.whfoods.com/genpage.php?tname=foodspice &dbid=97.

"Squash, Summer." World's Healthiest Foods. Accessed May 8, 2015. www.whfoods.com/genpage.php?tname=foodspice&dbid=62.

"Squash, Winter." World's Healthiest Foods. Accessed May 8, 2015. www.whfoods.com/genpage.php?tname=foodspice&dbid=63.

"How Many Vegetables Are Needed Daily or Weekly?" Choose My Plate. USDA. Accessed May 8, 2015. www.choosemyplate.gov /printpages/MyPlateFoodGroups/Vegetables/food-groups .vegetables-amount.pdf.

"Health Benefits of Citrus Fruit." Dairy Council of California. Accessed May 8, 2015. www.healthyeating.org/Healthy-Eating /All-Star-Foods/Fruits/Article-Viewer/Article/204/health -benefits-of-citrus-fruit.aspx.

Zelman, Kathleen M. "The Peach: 10 Healthy Facts"(July 8, 2010). www.webmd.com/food-recipes/peach-10-healthy-facts.

Vann, Madeline. "9 Amazing Health Benefits of Berries." Every- dayHealth.com. Accessed May 8, 2015. www.everydayhealth.com /diet-nutrition-pictures/amazing-health-benefits-of-berries.aspx.

"Grapes." World's Healthiest Foods. Accessed May 8, 2015. www.whfoods.com/genpage.php?tname=foodspice&dbid=40.

"Fresh, Frozen or Canned Fruits and Vegetables: All Can Be Healthy Choices!" American Heart Association. (Last modified June 25, 2015). www.heart.org/HEARTORG/GettingHealthy /NutritionCenter/SimpleCookingwithHeart/Fresh-Frozen-or -Canned-Fruits-and-Vegetables-All-Can-Be-Healthy-Choices _UCM_459350_Article.jsp.

"Fruits." ChooseMyPlate.gov. USDA. Accessed May 8, 2015. www.choosemyplate.gov/food-groups/fruits.html.

DRINK

"Medicines in My Home: Caffeine in Your Body." FDA, 2007. www.fda.gov/downloads/UCM200805.pdf.

Stromberg, Joseph. "This Is How Your Brain Becomes Addicted to Caffeine." *Smithsonian*, Aug. 9, 2013. www.smithsonianmag.com /science-nature/this-is-how-your-brain-becomes-addicted-to -caffeine-26861037/?no-ist.

Blakeslee, Sandra. "Yes, People Are Right. Caffeine Is Addictive." *The New York Times*, Oct. 4, 1994. www.nytimes.com/1994/10/05/ us/yes-people-are-right-caffeine-is-addictive.html.

Bushak, Lecia. "Fresh-Brewed Coffee May Act as an Antioxidant." *Medical Daily*, May 4, 2015. www.medicaldaily.com/health -benefits-coffee-caffeine-acts-antioxidant-fights-free-radicals -331856.

"What Are the Health Benefits of Coffee?" *Medical News Today*, Mar. 16, 2015. www.medicalnewstoday.com/articles/270202.php.

Pereira, M. A. "Coffee Consumption and Risk of Type 2 Diabetes Mellitus: An 11-Year Prospective Study of 28,812 Postmenopausal Women." *Archives of Internal Medicine* 166.12 (2006): 1311-16.

Saab, Sammy, Divya Mallam, Gerald A. Cox II, and Myron J. Tong. "Impact of Coffee on Liver Diseases: A Systematic Review." *Liver International* (2013).

"The Benefits of Caffeine on Motor Impairment in Parkinson's Disease." *Medical News Today*, Aug. 3, 2012. www.medicalnewstoday.com/releases/248568.php.

"Health Benefits Linked to Drinking Tea." *Harvard Health.* Accessed May 8, 2015. www.health.harvard.edu/press_releases /health-benefits-linked-to-drinking-tea.

Edgar, Julie. "Types of Tea and Their Health Benefits" (March 20, 2009). www.webmd.com/diet/tea-types-and-their-health -benefits.

"Learn About Alcohol: Signs Symptoms." National Council on Alcoholism and Drug Dependence. Accessed May 8, 2015. www.ncadd.org/learn-about-alcohol/signs-and-symptoms.

"Alcohol Withdrawal." MedlinePlus. U.S. National Library of Medicine. Accessed May 8, 2015. www.nlm.nih.gov/medlineplus /ency/article/000764.htm.

"Alcohol: Balancing Risks and Benefits." The Nutrition Source. Harvard T. H. Chan School of Public Health. Accessed May 8, 2015. www.hsph.harvard.edu/nutritionsource/alcohol-full-story/.

"Alcohol and Pregnancy." MedlinePlus. U.S. National Library of Medicine. Accessed May 8, 2015. www.nlm.nih.gov/medlineplus /ency/article/007454.htm.

"Alcohol Metabolism: An Update." National Institute of Alcoholism and Alcohol Abuse. Accessed May 8, 2015. www.pubs.niaaa .nih.gov/publications/AA72/AA72.htm.

Zahkari, Samir. "How Is Alcohol Metabolized in the Body." National Institute of Alcoholism and Alcohol Abuse. Accessed May 8, 2015. www.pubs.niaaa.nih.gov/publications/arh294 /245-255.pdf.

"Alcohol-Related Liver Disease." American Liver Foundation. Accessed May 8, 2015. www.liverfoundation.org/abouttheliver /info/alcohol/.

"Dehydration—Causes." UK National Health Service. Accessed May 8, 2015. www.nhs.uk/Conditions/Dehydration/Pages /Causes.aspx.

Suter, Paolo M., and Angelo Tremblay. "Is Alcohol Consumption a Risk Factor for Weight Gain and Obesity?" *Critical Reviews in Clinical Laboratory Sciences* 42.3 (2005): 197–227.

Nelson, Jennifer K. "Nutrition and Healthy Eating: Juicing: What Are the Health Benefits?" Mayo Clinic. Accessed May 8, 2015.

www.mayoclinic.org/healthy-lifestyle/nutrition-and-healthy -eating/expert-answers/juicing/faq-20058020.

"Abundance of Fructose Not Good for the Liver, Heart." *Harvard Health*, Sept. 1, 2011. www.health.harvard.edu/heart-health /abundance-of-fructose-not-good-for-the-liver-heart.

"Nonalcoholic Fatty Liver Disease." Mayo Clinic. Accessed May 8, 2015. www.mayoclinic.org/diseases-conditions/nonalcoholic -fatty-liver-disease/basics/definition/con-20027761.

"Baby Bottle Tooth Decay." Mouth Healthy. American Dental Association. Accessed May 8, 2015. www.mouthhealthy.org/en /az-topics/b/baby-bottle-tooth-decay.

DIETS

Atkins, Robert C. *Dr. Atkins' Diet Revolution: The High Calorie Way to Stay Thin Forever.* New York: Bantam, 1973.

Atkins, Robert C. *Dr. Atkins' New Diet Revolution.* New York: M. Evans, 2002.

"Myths and Facts of the Atkins Nutritional Approach." Atkins Nutritionals. Accessed May 8, 2015. www.atkins.com/how-it-works /library/articles/myths-and-facts-of-the-atkins-nutritional -approach.

Daly, M. E., R. Paisey, B. A. Millward, C. Eccles, et al. "Short-Term Effects of Severe Dietary Carbohydrate-Restriction Advice in Type 2 Diabetes—A Randomized Controlled Trial." *Diabetic Medicine* 23:1 (2006), 15–20.

"Low-Carbohydrate Diets." The Nutrition Source. Harvard T. H. Chan School of Public Health. Accessed May 8, 2015. www.hsph .harvard.edu/nutritionsource/carbohydrates/low-carbohydrate -diets/.

Halton, T. L., S. Liu, J. E. Manson, and F. B. Hu. "Low-Carbohydrate-Diet Score and Risk of Type 2 Diabetes in Women." *American Journal of Clinical Nutrition* 87:2 (2008), 339–46.

"Weight Loss: Atkins Diet: What's behind the Claims?" Mayo Clinic. Accessed May 8, 2015. www.mayoclinic.org/healthy -lifestyle/weight-loss/in-depth/atkins-diet/art-20048485.

"Raw Food Diet Overview." *U.S. News & World Report*. Accessed May 8, 2015. www.health.usnews.com/best-diet/raw-food-diet.

"What Is the Raw Food Diet? What Are the Benefits of the Raw Food Diet?" *Medical News Today*, Sept. 17, 2014. www.medicalnewstoday.com/articles/7381.php.

Ross, Robert Allan. "Raw Science: Why Alkalizing Food Is the Key to Life." Raw Food Life. Accessed May 8, 2015. www.rawfoodlife.com/#axzz3ZI6Lwu15.

Snyder, Kimberly. *The Beauty Detox Solution: Eat Your Way to Radiant Skin, Renewed Energy, and the Body You've Always Wanted*. Don Mills, Canada: Harlequin, 2011.

"Reality Check: 5 Risks of Raw Vegan Diet." Live Science. Accessed May 8, 2015. www.livescience.com/26278-risks-raw-vegan-diet.html.

Koebnick, Corinna, Ada Garcia, Pieter Dagnelie, Carola Strassner, et al. "Long-Term Consumption of a Raw Food Diet Is Associated with Favorable Serum LDL Cholesterol and Triglycerides but Also with Elevated Plasma Homocysteine and Low Serum HDL Cholesterol in Humans." *The Journal of Nutrition*, 2005. www.jn.nutrition.org/content/135/10/2372.long.

Moustapha, Ali, and Killian Robinson. "High Plasma Homocysteine: A Risk Factor for Vascular Disease in the Elderly." *Coronary Artery Disease* 9:11 (1998), 725–30.

"World History of Vegetarianism." *Vegetarian Society*. Accessed May 8, 2015. www.vegsoc.org/sslpage.aspx?pid=830.

"Why Go Vegan?" The Vegan Society. Accessed May 8, 2015. www.vegansociety.com/try-vegan/why-go-vegan.

"Could a Short Term Vegan Diet Improve Overall Health?" Food-Navigator.com. Accessed May 8, 2015. www.foodnavigator.com/Science/Could-a-short-term-vegan-diet-improve-overall-health.

Mcdougall, John, Laurie E. Thomas, Craig Mcdougall, Gavin Moloney, et al. "Effects of 7 Days on an Ad Libitum Low-Fat Vegan Diet: The McDougall Program Cohort." *Nutrition Journal* 13:1 (2014), 99.

Wheless, James W. "History of the Ketogenic Diet." *Epilepsia* 49 (2008), 3–5.

"Ketogenic Diet." Epilepsy Foundation. Accessed May 8, 2015. www.epilepsy.com/learn/treating-seizures-and-epilepsy/dietary-therapies/ketogenic-diet.

Sharman, M. J., W. J. Kraemer, D. M. Love, A. L. Gomez, et al. "A Ketogenic Diet Favorably Affects Serum Biomarkers for Cardiovascular Disease in Normal-Weight Men." *Journal of Nutrition* 132:7 (2002), 1879–85.

Meidenbauer, Joshua J., Nathan Ta, and Thomas Seyfried. "Influence of a Ketogenic Diet, Fish-Oil, and Calorie Restriction on Plasma Metabolites and Lipids in C57BL/6J Mice." *Nutrition & Metabolism* 2014. www.nutritionandmetabolism.com/content/11/1/23.

Dashti, Hussein M., Thazhumpal C. Mathew, Talib Hussein, Sami K. Asfar, et al. "Long-Term Effects of a Ketogenic Diet in Obese Patients." *Experimental & Clinical Cardiology*. Accessed May 8, 2015. www.ncbi.nlm.nih.gov/pmc/articles/PMC2716748/.

"Pros and Cons of the Paleo Diet." University of Pittsburgh Medical Center. Accessed May 8, 2015. www.upmc.com/services/sports-medicine/newsletter/pages/paleo-diet.aspx.

Frazier, Karen. *The Hashimoto's Diet and Action Plan*. Berkeley, CA: Rockridge, 2015.

Lindeberg, S., T. Jönsson, Y. Granfeldt, E. Borgstrand, J. Soffman, et al. "A Palaeolithic Diet Improves Glucose Tolerance More Than a Mediterranean-like Diet in Individuals with Ischaemic Heart Disease." *Diabetologia* 50:9 (2007), 1795–807.

Österdahl, M., T. Kocturk, A. Koochek, and P. E. Wändell. "Effects of a Short-Term Intervention with a Paleolithic Diet in Healthy Volunteers." *European Journal of Clinical Nutrition* 62:5 (2007), 682–85.

Jönsson, Tommy, Yvonne Granfeldt, Bo Ahrén, Ulla-Carin Branell, et al. "Beneficial Effects of a Paleolithic Diet on Cardiovascular Risk Factors in Type 2 Diabetes: A Randomized Cross-Over Pilot Study." *Cardiovascular Diabetology* 8:1 (2009), 35.

Frassetto, L. A., M. Schloetter, M. Mietus-Synder, R. C. Morris, and A. Sebastian. "Metabolic and Physiologic Improvements from Consuming a Paleolithic, Hunter-Gatherer Type Diet." *European Journal of Clinical Nutrition* 63:8 (2009), 947–55.

Ryberg, M., S. Sandberg, C. Mellberg, O. Stegle, et al. "A Paleolithic-Type Diet Causes Strong Tissue-Specific Effects on Ectopic Fat Deposition in Obese Postmenopausal Women." *Journal of Internal Medicine* 274:1 (2013), 67–76.

Mellberg, C., S. Sandberg, M. Ryberg, M. Eriksson, et al. "Long-Term Effects of a Palaeolithic-Type Diet in Obese Postmenopausal Women: A 2-Year Randomized Trial." *European Journal of Clinical Nutrition* 68 (2014): 350–57.

Bisht, Babita, Warren G. Darling, Ruth E. Grossmann, E. Torage Shivapour, et al. *The Journal of Alternative and Complementary Medicine* 20:5 (May 2014), 347–55. doi:10.1089/acm.2013.0188.

"Nutrition and Healthy Eating." Mediterranean Diet for Heart Health. Mayo Clinic. Accessed May 8, 2015. www.mayoclinic.org/healthy-lifestyle/nutrition-and-healthy-eating/in-depth/mediterranean-diet/art-20047801.

Altomare, Roberta, Francesco Cacciabaudo, Giuseppe Damiano, Vincenzo Davide Palumbo, et al. "The Mediterranean Diet: A History of Health." *Iranian Journal of Public Health.* Tehran University of Medical Sciences. www.ncbi.nlm.nih.gov/pmc/articles/PMC3684452/.

Palmer, Sharon. "The Mediterranean Diet—An Up-Close Look at Its Origins in Pantelleria." Today's Dietician, May 2013. www.todaysdietitian.com/newarchives/050113p28.shtml.

Goldman, Heidi. "Adopt a Mediterranean Diet Now for Better Health Later." Harvard Health Blog, Nov. 6, 2013. www.health.harvard.edu/blog/adopt-a-mediterranean-diet-now-for-better-health-later-201311066846.

"About Us." WeightWatchers.com. Accessed May 8, 2015. www.weightwatchers.com/about/prs/wwi_template.aspx?GCMSID=1002801.

Weaver, K. "Review: Little Evidence Supports the Efficacy of Major Commercial and Organised Self Help Weight Loss Programmes." *Evidence-Based Nursing* 8:3 (2005), 77.

Muzio, F., L. Mondazzi, D. Sommariva, and A. Branchi. "Long-Term Effects of Low-Calorie Diet on the Metabolic Syndrome in Obese Nondiabetic Patients." *Diabetes Care* 28:6 (2005), 1485–86.

Vansant, G., L. Van Gaal, and I. Dee Leuw. "Short and Long Term Effects of a Very Low Calorie Diet on Resting Metabolic Rate and Body Composition." *International Journal of Obesity* 13, Suppl, 2 (1989), 87–9. *PubMed.*

"Nutrition and Healthy Eating." Mayo Clinic. Accessed May 8, 2015. www.mayoclinic.org/healthy-lifestyle/nutrition-and-healthy-eating/in-depth/dash-diet/art-20048456.

"What Is the DASH Eating Plan?" National Heart, Lung, and Blood Institute. Accessed May 8, 2015. www.nhlbi.nih.gov/health/health-topics/topics/dash.

"Compared with Usual Sodium Intake, Low- and Excessive-Sodium Diets Are Associated with Increased Mortality: A Meta-Analysis." *American Journal of Hypertension* 27:9 (Sept. 2014), 1129–37. doi:10.1093/ajh/hpu028.

Svetkey, L. P. "Effects of Dietary Patterns on Blood Pressure: Subgroup Analysis of the Dietary Approaches to Stop Hypertension (DASH) Randomized Clinical Trial." *Archives of Internal Medicine* 159:3 (1999), 285–93.

Moore, Thomas J., Paul R. Conlin, Jamy Ard, and Laura P. Svetsky. "DASH (Dietary Approaches to Stop Hypertension) Diet Is Effective Treatment for Stage 1 Isolated Systolic Hypertension." *Hypertension* 38 (2001): 155–8.

"Food Safety for Moms-to-Be: Safe Eats—Fruits, Veggies & Juices." FDA. Accessed May 8, 2015. www.fda.gov/Food/ResourcesForYou/HealthEducators/ucm081785.htm.

"Climate Change and Nutrition." London School of Hygiene and Tropical Medicine. Accessed May 8, 2015. www.ble.lshtm.ac.uk/pluginfile.php/20037/mod_resource/content/43/OER/PNO101/sessions/S1S13/PNO101_S1S13_040_010.html.

ADDITIONAL REFERENCES

Doheny, Kathleen. "'Grazing' Appears No Better for Weight Loss Than Standard Meals." Health Day, Mar. 27, 2014. www.consumer.healthday.com/vitamins-and-nutrition-information-27

/dieting-to-lose-weight-health-news-195/grazing-no-better-for-weight-control-than-standard-meals-study-686150.html.

Hites, R. A. "Global Assessment of Organic Contaminants in Farmed Salmon." *Science* 303:5655 (2004), 226–29. DOI: 10.1126/science.1091447.

Bastin, Sandra. "Preserving Nutrients in Food." University of Kentucky. Accessed May 8, 2015. www2.ca.uky.edu/hes/fcs/factshts/FN-SSB.006.PDF.

CHAPTER FIVE: AILMENTS & ALLERGIES

AILMENTS

Koufman, Jamie, Jordan Stern, and Marc Bauer. *Dropping Acid: The Reflux Diet Cookbook & Cure*. New York: Reflux Cook, 2010.

Kern, Daniel W. "Diet and Acne." Acne.org. Accessed May 8, 2015. www.acne.org/diet.html.

Aubrey, Alison. "Diet and Acne: For a Clearer Complexion, Cut the Empty Carbs." NPR, Feb. 20, 2013. www.npr.org/blogs/thesalt/2013/02/19/172429086/diet-and-acne-for-a-clearer-complexion-cut-the-empty-carbs.

Klein, Sarah. "Inflammatory Foods: 9 of the Worst Picks for Inflammation." TheHuffingtonPost.com, Mar. 21, 2013. www.huffingtonpost.com/2013/03/21/inflammatory-foods-worst-inflammation_n_2838643.html.

"Acne Basics." Mayo Clinic. Accessed May 8, 2015. www.mayoclinic.org/diseases-conditions/acne/basics/causes/con-20020580.

Clark, Nancy. "Nutrition Advice for Active Women with Amenorrhea." College of Agriculture and Life Sciences. North Carolina State University. Accessed May 8, 2015. www.cals.ncsu.edu/course/ntr301/AMNRRHA.HTM.

"Anemia." Diseases and Conditions. Mayo Clinic. Accessed May 8, 2015. www.mayoclinic.org/diseases-conditions/anemia/basics/definition/con-20026209.

"Vitamins," MedlinePlus. U.S. National Library of Medicine. Accessed May 8, 2015. www.nlm.nih.gov/medlineplus/ency/article/002399.htm.

"Anemia and Nutrition: The Importance of Essential Vitamins." Anemia.org, Oct. 9, 2008. Accessed May 8, 2015. www.anemia.org/patients/feature-articles/content.php?contentid=000275.

"Three of the B Vitamins: Folate, Vitamin B_6, and Vitamin B_{12}." The Nutrition Source. Harvard School of Public Health. Accessed May 8, 2015. www.hsph.harvard.edu/nutritionsource/vitamin-b/.

"Depression and Anxiety: Nutritional Considerations." Physicians' Committee for Responsible Medicine. Accessed May 8, 2015. www.nutritionmd.org/health_care_providers/psychiatric/depression_nutrition.html.

"Anti-Inflammatory Diet for Arthritis." Arthritis Foundation. Accessed May 8, 2015. www.arthritis.org/living-with-arthritis/arthritis-diet/anti-inflammatory/.

"Anti-Inflammatory Diet." Arthritis Foundation. Accessed May 8, 2015. www.arthritis.org/living-with-arthritis/arthritis-diet/anti-inflammatory/anti-inflammatory-diet.php.

"High Cooking Temperature and Inflammation." Arthritis Foundation. Accessed May 8, 2015. www.arthritis.org/living-with-arthritis/arthritis-diet/anti-inflammatory/cooking-temperature-inflammatiohp.

"Foods That Fight Inflammation." Arthritis Foundation. Accessed May 8, 2015. www.arthritis.org/living-with-arthritis/arthritis-diet/anti-inflammatory/eat-to-beat-inflammation.php.

"More Fiber, Less Inflammation?" Arthritis Foundation. Accessed May 8, 2015. www.arthritis.org/living-with-arthritis/arthritis-diet/anti-inflammatory/fiber-inflammation.php.

"ADHD Diets for Children and Adults." WebMD. Accessed May 8, 2015. www.webmd.com/add-adhd/guide/adhd-diets.

"Diet and Attention Deficit Hyperactivity Disorder." Harvard Health. Harvard Medical School. Accessed May 8, 2015. www.health.harvard.edu/newsletter_article/Diet-and-attention-deficit-hyperactivity-disorder.

"Gluten Free/Casein Free Diets for Autism." WebMD. Accessed May 8, 2015. www.webmd.com/brain/autism/gluten-free-casein-free-diets-for-autism.

"Autoimmune Diseases, " MedlinePlus. U.S. National Library of Medicine. Accessed May 8, 2015. www.nlm.nih.gov/medlineplus/autoimmunediseases.html.

"Anti-Inflammatory Diet Fact Sheet." Sjorgrens Syndrome Foundation. Accessed May 8, 2015. www.sjogrens.org/files/brochures/anti-inflammatory_diet.pdf.

Hendon, Louise. "The Definitive Guide to the Paleo Autoimmune Protocol (AIP)." *Paleo Living Magazine*, Feb. 3, 2014. www.paleomagazine.com/definitive-guide-to-the-paleo-autoimmune-protocol-aip/.

Blum, Susan S., and Michele Bender. *The Immune System Recovery Plan: A Doctor's 4-step Program to Treat Autoimmune Disease.* New York: Scribner, 2013.

"Muscle Spasms/Cramps: Nutritional Treatment, Causes, Remedies, Prevention." ACU Cell Disorders. Accessed May 8, 2015. www.acu-cell.com/dis-mus.html.

"Food for Thought: Diet and Nutrition for a Healthy Back." Veritas Health. Accessed May 8, 2015. www.spine-health.com/wellness/nutrition-diet-weight-loss/food-thought-diet-and-nutrition-a-healthy-back.

Weil, Andrew. "Condition Care Guide." *Dr. Andrew Weil.* Accessed May 8, 2015. www.drweil.com/drw/u/ART02931/Bruises.html.

Whitaker, Julian. "Treatments for Easily Bruised Skin." *Dr. Julian Whitaker.* Accessed May 8, 2015. www.drwhitaker.com/treatments-for-easily-bruised-skin.

"Vitamin K." U.S. National Library of Medicine. Accessed May 8, 2015. www.nlm.nih.gov/medlineplus/ency/article/002407.htm.

"Once Treatment Starts." American Cancer Society. Accessed May 8, 2015. www.cancer.org/treatment/survivorship duringandaftertreatment/nutritionforpeoplewithcancer/nutritionforthepersonwithcancer/nutrition-during-treatment-once-treatment-starts.

"What Is Celiac Disease?" Celiac Disease Foundation. Accessed May 8, 2015. www.celiac.org/celiac-disease/what-is-celiac-disease/.

"Celiac Disease," MedlinePlus. U.S. National Library of Medicine. Accessed May 8, 2015. www.nlm.nih.gov/medlineplus/ency/article/002443.htm.

"Cold Sores (HSV-1)." KidsHealth. Ed. Mary L. Gavin. The Nemours Foundation, Feb. 1, 2014. www.kidshealth.org/teen/your_body/skin_stuff/cold_sores.html.

"Diet and Nutrition with Herpes." Herpes Support Network. Accessed May 8, 2015. www.herpes-coldsores.com/diet_and_nutrition_with_herpes.htm.

"Cold Sore." Alternative Medicine. Mayo Clinic. Accessed May 8, 2015. www.mayoclinic.org/diseases-conditions/cold-sore/basics/alternative-medicine/con-20021310.

Weil, Andrew. "Condition Care Guide." *Dr. Andrew Weil.* Accessed May 8, 2015. www.drweil.com/drw/u/ART00372/Herpes-Treatment.html.

"Starve a Cold, Feed a Fever? Learn the Facts." WebMD. Accessed May 8, 2015. www.webmd.com/cold-and-flu/cold-guide/starve-cold-feed-fever.

"Chicken Soup: Can It Cure a Cold?" Diseases and Conditions. Mayo Clinic. Accessed May 8, 2015. www.mayoclinic.org/diseases-conditions/common-cold/in-depth/health-tip/art-20048631.

"Constipation." Diseases and Conditions. Mayo Clinic. Accessed May 8, 2015. www.mayoclinic.org/diseases-conditions/constipation/basics/definition/con-20032773.

"Eating, Diet, and Nutrition for Constipation." National Institutes of Health. Accessed May 8, 2015. www.niddk.nih.gov/health-information/health-topics/digestive-diseases/constipation/Pages/eating-diet-nutrition.aspx.

"Constipation." The Cleveland Clinic. Accessed May 8, 2015. www.my.clevelandclinic.org/health/diseases_conditions/hic_constipation.

Hyman, Mark. "Magnesium: Meet the Most Powerful Relaxation Mineral Available." DrHyman.com, Oct. 19, 2014. www.drhyman.com/blog/2010/05/20/magnesium-the-most-powerful-relaxation-mineral-available/.

Breyer, Melissa. "10 Natural Cough Remedies." Mother Nature Network, Dec. 12, 2013. www.mnn.com/health/fitness-well-being/stories/10-natural-cough-remedies.

"Is There a Dandruff Diet?" WebMD. Accessed May 8, 2015. www.webmd.com/skin-problems-and-treatments/dandruff-13/food-link.

Dale, Nick. "Perth Naturopath." Perth Naturopath. Accessed May 8, 2015. www.perth-naturopath.com/nutritional-deificiencies.html.

Rao, T. S. Sathyanarayana, M. R. Asha, B. N. Ramesh, and K. S. Jagannatha Rao. "Understanding Nutrition, Depression and Mental Illnesses." *Indian Journal of Psychiatry*. Accessed May 8, 2015. www.ncbi.nlm.nih.gov/pmc/articles/PMC2738337/.

Hall-Flavin, Daniel K. "Vitamin B-12 and Depression: Are They Related?" Ask an Expert. Mayo Clinic, accessed May 8, 2015. www.mayoclinic.org/diseases-conditions/depression/expert-answers/vitamin-b12-and-depression/faq-20058077.

"Type 2 Diabetes." The Nutrition Source. Harvard T. H. Chan School of Public Health. Accessed May 8, 2015. www.hsph.harvard.edu/nutritionsource/type-2-diabetes/.

"Diabetes Type 2—Meal Planning." U.S. National Library of Medicine. Accessed May 8, 2015. www.nlm.nih.gov/medlineplus/ency/article/007429.htm.

Davis, N. J., N. Tomuta, C. Schechter, C. R. Isasi, et al. "Comparative Study of the Effects of a 1-Year Dietary Intervention of a Low-Carbohydrate Diet Versus a Low-Fat Diet on Weight and Glycemic Control in Type 2 Diabetes." *Diabetes Care* 32:7 (2009), 1147–52.

"BRAT Diet: Recovering From an Upset Stomach." American Academy of Family Physicians Foundation. Accessed May 8, 2015. www.familydoctor.org/familydoctor/en/prevention-wellness/food-nutrition/weight-loss/brat-diet-recovering-from-an-upset-stomach.html.

"When You Have Diarrhea." U.S. National Library of Medicine. Accessed May 8, 2015. www.nlm.nih.gov/medlineplus/ency/patientinstructions/000121.htm.

"Using Foods Against Menstrual Pain." Physicians' Committee for Responsible Medicine. Accessed May 8, 2015. www.pcrm.org/health/health-topics/using-foods-against-menstrual-pain.

"Eczema." University of Maryland. Accessed May 8, 2015. www.umm.edu/health/medical/altmed/condition/eczema.

Veracity, Daniel. "The Hidden Dangers of Caffeine: How Coffee Causes Exhaustion, Fatigue and Addiction." Natural News Network, Oct. 11, 2005. www.naturalnews.com/012352_caffeine_coffee.html#ixzz3ZZOq3ez1.

Fischetti, Mark. "Fact or Fiction?: Feed a Cold, Starve a Fever." *Scientific American*, Jan. 3, 2014. www.scientificamerican.com/article/fact-or-fiction-feed-a-cold/.

"Fibromyalgia: The Diet Connection." MedicineNet. Accessed May 8, 2015. www.medicinenet.com/script/main/art.asp?articlekey=104485.

"Fibromyalgia." University of Maryland. Accessed May 8, 2015. www.umm.edu/health/medical/reports/articles/fibromyalgia.

"Food Poisoning." Diseases and Conditions. Mayo Clinic. Accessed May 8, 2015. www.mayoclinic.org/diseases-conditions/food-poisoning/basics/symptoms/con-20031705.

Watson, Stephanie. "Gallbladder Diet: Foods for Gallbladder Problems." WebMD. Accessed May 8, 2015. www.webmd.com/digestive-disorders/features/gallbladder-diet-foods-for-gallbadder-problems.

"Gallbladder Disease." University of Maryland Medical Center, www.umm.edu/health/medical/altmed/condition/gallbladder-disease. Accessed 23 May 2015.

"Gas and Gas Pains." Mayo Clinic. Accessed May 8, 2015. www.mayoclinic.org/diseases-conditions/gas-and-gas-pains/in-depth/gas-and-gas-pains/art-20044739

"Viral Gastroenteritis (Stomach Flu)." Diseases and Conditions. Mayo Clinic. Accessed May 8, 2015. www.mayoclinic.org /diseases-conditions/viral-gastroenteritis/basics/definition /con-20019350.

"Gout Diet: What's Allowed, What's Not." Nutrition and Healthy Eating. Mayo Clinic. Accessed May 8, 2015. www.mayoclinic.org /healthy-lifestyle/nutrition-and-healthy-eating/in-depth/gout -diet/art-20048524.

"Hair Loss." Diseases and Conditions. Mayo Clinic. Accessed May 8, 2015. www.mayoclinic.org/diseases-conditions/hair-loss /basics/definition/con-20027666.

"Vitamin B$_5$, Pantothenic Acid, Vitamin B$_5$ Acne, Pantothenic Acid Benefits, Vitamin B$_5$ Foods." DMS Nutrition Products Europe. Accessed May 8, 2015. www.nutri-facts.org/eng/vitamins /vitamin-b5-pantothenic-acid/at-a-glance/.

"9 Foods That Fight Bad Breath." Mother Nature Network. Accessed May 8, 2015. www.mnn.com/food/healthy-eating /stories/9-foods-that-fight-bad-breath.

"Breath Odor." National Institute of Health. www.nlm.nih.gov /medlineplus/ency/article/003058.htm.

"Headache Suffer's Diet." National Headache Foundation. Accessed May 23, 2015. www.headaches.org/headache-sufferers -diet.

"Tyramine-Rich Foods: Do They Trigger Migraines?" WebMD. Accessed May 8, 2015. www.webmd.com/migraines-headaches /guide/tyramine-and-migraines.

"Identifying Food Triggers for Migraines." *WebMD*. WebMD. Accessed May 8, 2015. www.webmd.com/migraines-headaches /features/identifying-food-triggers-for-migraines?page=2.

"About Cholesterol." American Heart Association. Accessed May 8, 2015. www.heart.org/HEARTORG/Conditions/Cholesterol /AboutCholesterol/About-Cholesterol_UCM_001220_Article.jsp.

"11 Foods That Lower Cholesterol." Harvard Health. Harvard Medical School. Accessed May 8, 2015. www.health.harvard.edu /heart-health/11-foods-that-lower-cholesterol.

"13 Power Foods That Lower Blood Pressure Naturally." *Prevention*. Accessed May 8, 2015. www.prevention.com/food/13-power -foods-lower-blood-pressure-naturally.

"10 Ways to Control High Blood Pressure without Medication." Diseases and Conditions. Mayo Clinic. Accessed May 8, 2015. www.mayoclinic.org/diseases-conditions/high-blood-pressure /in-depth/high-blood-pressure/art-20046974.

Weil, Andrew. "High Blood Pressure Treatment." *Dr. Andrew Weil*. Accessed May 8, 2015. www.drweil.com/drw/u/ART00686 /high-blood-pressure-treatment.

"Low Blood Pressure (Hypotension)." Diseases and Conditions. Mayo Clinic. Accessed May 8, 2015. www.mayoclinic.org /diseases-conditions/low-blood-pressure/basics/definition /con-20032298.

"Eating Can Cause Low Blood Pressure." Harvard Health. Harvard Medical School. Accessed May 8, 2015. www.health.harvard. edu/heart-health/eating-can-cause-low-blood-pressure.

"Hyperthyroidism Overview." Vertical Health. Accessed May 8, 2015. www.endocrineweb.com/conditions/hyperthyroidism /hyperthyroidism-overview-overactive-thyroid.

"5 Foods That May Help Ease Hyperthyroidism Symptoms." Vertical Health. Accessed May 8, 2015. www.endocrineweb.com /conditions/hyperthyroidism/5-foods-may-help-ease -hyperthyroidism-symptoms.

Pick, Marcelle. "Thyroid Health and Selenium." Women to Women. Accessed May 8, 2015. www.womentowomen.com /thyroid-health/thyroid-health-and-selenium/.

Kresser, Chris. "Selenium: The Missing Link for Treating Hypothyroidism?" Feb. 3, 2012. www.chriskresser.com/selenium -the-missing-link-for-treating-hypothyroidism/.

Drutel, Anne, Françoise Archambeaud, and Philippe Caron. "Selenium and the Thyroid Gland: More Good News for Clinicians." *Clinical Endocrinology* 78:2 (2013), 155–64.

"The Monash University Low FODMAP Diet." Monash University. Accessed May 8, 2015. www.med.monash.edu/cecs/gastro /fodmap/low-high.html.

"What Is Inflammation?" U.S. National Library of Medicine. Accessed May 8, 2015. www.ncbi.nlm.nih.gov/pubmedhealth /PMH0072482/.

Weil, Andrew. "Anti-Inflammatory Diet & Pyramid." *Dr. Andrew Weil*. Accessed May 8, 2015. www.drweil.com/drw/u/ART02995 /Dr-Weil-Anti-Inflammatory-Food-Pyramid.html.

"How Foods Can Affect Your Immunity to the Flu." National Institute of Allergy and Infectious Diseases. National Institutes of Health, Feb. 27, 2007. www.niaid.nih.gov/topics/Flu/Research /vaccineResearch/Pages/foodsAffectImmunity.aspx.

Young, Allison. "Exactly What to Eat When You Have a Cold or Flu." *Prevention*, Jan. 8, 2015. www.prevention.com/health /health-concerns/what-eat-when-sick.

"Natural Sleep Solutions." WebMD. Accessed May 8, 2015. www.webmd.com/sleep-disorders/living-with-insomnia-11 /natural-solutions?page=2.

Peri, Camille. "RA and Diet: Foods to Eat to Beat Inflammation, Joint Pain, and Fatigue." WebMD. Accessed May 8, 2015. www.webmd.com/rheumatoid-arthritis/features/ra-diet.

"Diet and Kidney Stones." National Kidney Foundation. Accessed May 8, 2015. www.kidney.org/atoz/content/diet.

"Kidney Stones." Diseases and Conditions. Mayo Clinic. Accessed May 8, 2015. www.mayoclinic.org/diseases-conditions/kidney -stones/basics/definition/con-20024829?utm_source=Google &utm_medium=abstract&utm_content=Kidney-stone&utm _campaign=Knowledge-panel.

Firger, Jessica. "What Causes Leg Cramps and How Can You Stop Them?" Everyday Health Media. Accessed May 8, 2015. www.everydayhealth.com/pain-management/what-causes-leg -cramps-and-how-can-you-stop-them.aspx.

Pick, Marcelle. "Nutritional Relief for Hot Flashes." Women to Women. Accessed May 8, 2015. www.womentowomen.com /menopause-perimenopause/nutritional-relief-for-hot-flashes/.

"Menopause and Osteoporosis." Diseases and Conditions. Cleveland Clinic. Accessed May 8, 2015. www.my.clevelandclinic.org /health/diseases_conditions/hic-what-is-perimenopause -menopause-postmenopause/hic_Menopause_and _Osteoporosis.

"Osteoporosis." Diseases and Conditions. Mayo Clinic. Accessed May 8, 2015. www.mayoclinic.org/diseases-conditions /osteoporosis/basics/definition/con-20019924.

"Food and Your Bones." National Osteoporosis Foundation. Accessed May 8, 2015. www.nof.org/foods.

Glassman, Keri. "18 Foods That Help Fight PMS." *Women's Health Magazine*, May 22, 2014. www.womenshealthmag.com /nutrition/foods-fight-pms.

"PMS: Diet Dos and Don'ts." WebMD. Accessed May 8, 2015. www.webmd.com/women/pms/features/diet-and-pms?page=2.

"Enlarged Prostate." U.S. National Library of Medicine. Accessed May 8, 2015. www.nlm.nih.gov/medlineplus/ency/article /000381.htm.

"10 Diet & Exercise Tips for Prostate Health." Harvard Health. Harvard Medical School. Accessed May 8, 2015. www.health .harvard.edu/healthbeat/10-diet-and-exercise-tips-for -prostate-health.

"A New Diet to Quash Inflammation May Benefit Men's Prostate Health." Prostate Research Foundation, June 20, 2013. www.pcf .org/site/c.leJRIROrEpH/b.8723169/k.5845/A_New_Diet_to _Quash_Inflammation_May_Benefit_Men8217s_Prostate _Health.htm.

"Fast Facts About Psoriasis." National Institute of Arthritis and Musculoskeletal and Skin Disease. National Institutes of Health. Accessed May 8, 2015.

"Nutrition and Psoriatic Disease." Psoriatic Disease. National Psoriasis Foundation. Accessed May 8, 2015.

"Psoriasis: Nutritional Considerations." NutritionMD.org. Physicians' Committee for Responsible Medicine. Accessed May 8, 2015.

"All About Rosacea." All About Rosacea. National Rosacea Society. Accessed May 8, 2015. www.rosacea.org/patients /allaboutrosacea.php.

"Factors That May Trigger Rosacea Flare-Ups." National Rosacea Society. Accessed May 8, 2015. www.rosacea.org/patients/materials/triggers.php.

Melone, Linda. "Best and Worst Foods to Eat When Sick." Cable News Network, Mar. 31, 2015. www.cnn.com/2015/03/31/health/best-and-worst-foods-to-eat-sick/.

Davis, Sarah. "What to Eat When You Have a Sore Throat." Livestrong.com, Feb. 21, 2014. www.livestrong.com/article/96350-things-eat-sore-throat/.

"Drugs, Food and Drink." BTA. British Tinnitus Association. Accessed May 8, 2015. www.tinnitus.org.uk/drugs-food-and-drink.

"General Wellness." American Tinnitus Association. Accessed May 8, 2015. www.ata.org/managing-your-tinnitus/treatment-options/general-wellness.

"Stomach and Duodenal Ulcers (Peptic Ulcers)." Johns Hopkins Medical Center. Accessed May 8, 2015. www.hopkinsmedicine.org/healthlibrary/conditions/digestive_disorders/stomach_and_duodenal_ulcers_peptic_ulcers_85,P00394/.

Weil, Andrew. "Ulcers, Peptic Ulcer Disease (PUD)." *Dr. Andrew Weil*. Accessed May 8, 2015. www.drweil.com/drw/u/ART03201/Ulcers-Peptic-Ulcer-Disease-PUD.html.

"Urinary Tract Infection in Women." University of Maryland. Accessed May 8, 2015. umm.edu/health/medical/altmed/condition/urinary-tract-infection-in-women.

Elnima, El, S. A. Ahmed, A. G. Mekkawi, and J. S. Mossa. "The Antimicrobial Activity of Garlic and Onion Extracts." *Pharmazie* 38:11 (1993), 747–8.

"Urinary Tract Infections (UTIs)." Johns Hopkins Medical Center. Accessed May 8, 2015. www.hopkinsmedicine.org/healthlibrary/conditions/kidney_and_urinary_system_disorders/urinary_tract_infections_utis_85,P01497/.

"How to Prevent Yeast Infections." WebMD. Accessed May 8, 2015. www.webmd.com/women/10-ways-to-prevent-yeast-infections.

FOOD ALLERGIES

"What Is Food Allergy?" National Institute of Allergy and Infectious Diseases. National Institutes of Health. Accessed May 8, 2015. www.niaid.nih.gov/topics/foodallergy/understanding/pages/whatisit.aspx.

"What Is an Allergic Reaction to Food?" National Institute of Allergy and Infectious Diseases. National Institutes of Health. Accessed May 8, 2015. www.niaid.nih.gov/topics/foodAllergy/understanding/Pages/allergicRxn.aspx.

"Food Allergy vs. Food Intolerance: What's the Difference?" National Institute of Allergy and Infectious Diseases. National Institutes of Health. Accessed May 8, 2015. www.mayoclinic.org/diseases-conditions/food-allergy/expert-answers/food-allergy/faq-20058538.

"Peanut—Food Allergy Research & Education." National Institute of Allergy and Infectious Diseases. National Institutes of Health. Accessed May 8, 2015. www.foodallergy.org/allergens/peanut-allergy.

"'Outgrown' a Peanut Allergy? Eat More Peanuts!" National Institute of Allergy and Infectious Diseases. National Institutes of Health. Accessed May 8, 2015. www.hopkinsmedicine.org/press_releases/2004/11_09a_04.html.

Sircherer, S. H., A. Munoz-Furlong, and H. A. Sampson. "Prevalence of Peanut and Tree Nut Allergy in the United States Determined by Means of a Random Digit Dial Telephone Survey: A 5-Year Follow-Up Study." *Journal of Allergy and Clinical Immunology* 112:6 (2003), 1203–7.

"Tree Nut Allergy—Food Allergy Research & Education." National Institute of Allergy and Infectious Diseases. National Institutes of Health. Accessed May 8, 2015. www.foodallergy.org/allergens/tree-nut-allergy.

"Milk Allergy—Food Allergy Research & Education." National Institute of Allergy and Infectious Diseases. National Institutes of Health. Accessed May 8, 2015. www.foodallergy.org/allergens/milk-allergy.

"Egg—Food Allergy Research & Education." National Institute of Allergy and Infectious Diseases. National Institutes of Health. Accessed May 8, 2015. www.foodallergy.org/allergens/egg-allergy.

"Wheat—Food Allergy Research & Education." National Institute of Allergy and Infectious Diseases. National Institutes of Health. Accessed May 8, 2015. www.foodallergy.org/allergens/wheat -allergy.

"Fish—Food Allergy Research & Education." National Institute of Allergy and Infectious Diseases. National Institutes of Health. Accessed May 8, 2015. www.foodallergy.org/allergens/fish-allergy.

"Soy—Food Allergy Research & Education." National Institute of Allergy and Infectious Diseases. National Institutes of Health. Accessed May 8, 2015. www.foodallergy.org/allergens/soy-allergy.

Laino, Charlene. "Sesame Allergies on the Rise in U.S." WebMD. WebMD, Mar. 16, 2009. www.webmd.com/allergies/news /20090316/sesame-allergies-on-the-rise-in-us.

"Celery Allergy—the Facts." Anaphylaxis Campaign. Accessed May 8, 2015. www.anaphylaxis.org.uk/what-is-anaphylaxis /knowledgebase/celery-allergy--the-facts?page=3.

ADDITIONAL REFERENCES

"Lowering Salt in Your Diet." U.S. Food and Drug Administration. Accessed May 8, 2015. www.fda.gov/ForConsumers /ConsumerUpdates/ucm181577.htm.

Caldwell, Emily. "Study: Doubling Saturated Fat in the Diet Does Not Increase Saturated Fat in Blood." Nov. 21, 2014. www.news. osu.edu/news/2014/11/21/study-doubling-saturated-fat-in-the -diet-does-not-increase-saturated-fat-in-blood/.

"Study Shows No Association between Dietary Saturated Fats and Cardiovascular Disease Risk." European Union Food Information Council. Accessed May 8, 2015. www.eufic.org/page/en /show/latest-science-news/fftid/Study-no-association-dietary -saturated-fats-cardiovascular-disease-risk/.

Corliss, Julie. "Eating Too Much Added Sugar Increases the Risk of Dying with Heart Disease." Harvard Health Blog, Feb. 6, 2014. www.health.harvard.edu/blog/eating-too-much-added-sugar -increases-the-risk-of-dying-with-heart-disease-201402067021.

"Why Must Some Medicines Be Taken with or after Food?" UK National Health Service. Accessed May 8, 2015. www.nhs.uk/chq /Pages/866.aspx?CategoryID=73.

APPENDIX A: HOW TO READ A NUTRITION LABEL

"Food Labeling Guide." U.S. Food and Drug Administration, accessed May 8, 2015. www.fda.gov/Food/GuidanceRegulation /GuidanceDocumentsRegulatoryInformation/LabelingNutrition /ucm2006828.htm.

"How to Understand and Use the Nutrition Facts Label." U.S. Food and Drug Administration. www.fda.gov/Food /IngredientsPackagingLabeling/LabelingNutrition/ucm274593 .htm. Accessed May 23, 2015.

index

CPSIA information can be obtained
at www.ICGtesting.com
Printed in the USA
JSHW010823240721
17139JS00001B/1